5-MINUTE
YOGA

5-MINUTE

YOGA

A More Energetic, Focused, and Balanced You
in Just 5 MINUTES A DAY

Adams Media
New York   London   Toronto   Sydney   New Delhi

Adamsmedia

Adams Media
An Imprint of Simon & Schuster, Inc.
57 Littlefield Street
Avon, Massachusetts 02322

First Adams Media trade paperback edition JANUARY 2018

ADAMS MEDIA and colophon are trademarks of Simon and Schuster.

For information about special discounts for bulk purchases, please contact Simon & Schuster Special Sales at 1-866-506-1949 or business@simonandschuster.com.

The Simon & Schuster Speakers Bureau can bring authors to your live event. For more information or to book an event contact the Simon & Schuster Speakers Bureau at 1-866-248-3049 or visit our website at www.simonspeakers.com.

Interior design by Michelle Kelly
Interior illustrations by Eric Andrews

Manufactured in the United States of America

10 9 8 7 6 5 4 3 2 1

Library of Congress Cataloging-in-Publication Data has been applied for.

ISBN 978-1-5072-0632-4
ISBN 978-1-5072-0633-1 (ebook)

Contains material adapted from the following title published by Adams Media, an Imprint of Simon & Schuster, Inc.: *My Pocket Yoga* by Adams Media, copyright © 2017, ISBN 978-1-4405-9944-6.

CONTENTS

INTRODUCTION

Whether you love yoga but can't find time to get to a class regularly or just want to try a few poses at home, *5-Minute Yoga* is here to help. Yoga can help you strengthen your body, quiet and focus your mind, relieve tension, increase your awareness, improve your quality of life, and change how you see the world. It truly has a profound and lasting effect on how you treat yourself and others. Time spent doing yoga is an opportunity to focus on yourself completely and to reconnect with yourself on many levels.

If you are like most people, you just don't have time for an hour-long yoga class at a studio across town. Instead, you need simple, quick ways to incorporate yoga into your life. With that in mind, each of the one hundred sequences in this book incorporates basic yoga poses that together can be completed in just 5 minutes or less. Whether you're looking to boost your energy levels, find inner peace, lose weight, or strengthen your focus, you'll find easy sequences in this book that will improve your life—physically and spiritually.

5-Minute Yoga will help you become centered, calm, rejuvenated, and better able to face life's challenges, big and small—5 minutes at a time.

SEQUENCES
MIND

YOGA SEQUENCES FOR FOCUS

So many things in the modern world compete for our attention. Let yoga help you strengthen your ability to shut out distractions and put your mind back in charge of your attention. After doing just one of these sequences, you will find yourself better able to concentrate on the tasks ahead.

Focus Sequence 1

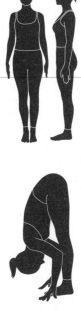

1. **Mountain Pose:** Stand tall, inhale, and reach your arms straight up to the ceiling. Ground down through the soles of your feet and squeeze your inner thighs together. Keep your lower ribs in and turn your pinkies inward to relax your shoulders away from your ears. Take 10 full breaths (1 minute). Return your arms to your sides.

2. **Standing Forward Bend:** Exhale and hinge at your hips. Let your torso drape over your thighs and reach your fingers toward the ground, bending as far as you can comfortably to release your lower back. Take 3 full breaths (15 seconds).

3. **Plank Pose:** Exhale, plant your hands palms down, shoulder-width apart, and extend your legs behind you. Place your feet hip-width apart with your toes pointed down. Create one long line of energy from your heels to the top of your head. Inhale.

4. **Cat-Cow:** Exhale and drop down to your hands and knees. Inhale, drop your belly, and arch your back, raising your tailbone. Lift your gaze as you find expansion across your chest. Exhale, arch your spine up, and lower your tailbone. Let your head hang heavy and look down between your thighs. Take 10 full breaths (1 minute).

5. **Bound Angle Pose:** Sit up tall on your mat. Bring the soles of your feet together in front of you and let your knees drop out to the sides. Hold your feet in your hands and pull them in toward your inner thighs as far as you can comfortably. Bring your arms in flat against your torso and place your fingertips on the mat behind your hips. Take 20 full breaths (2 minutes).

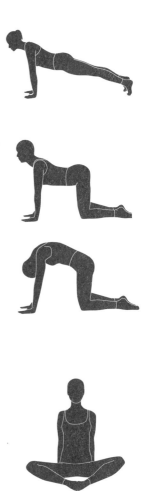

Focus Sequence 2

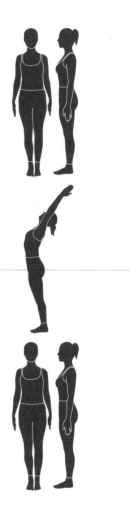

1. **Mountain Pose:** Stand tall, inhale, and reach your arms straight up to the ceiling. Ground down through the soles of your feet and squeeze your inner thighs together. Keep your lower ribs in and turn your pinkies inward to relax your shoulders away from your ears. Take 10 full breaths (1 minute). Return your arms to your sides.

2. **Standing Backbend Pose:** Exhale, bring your palms together over your head, and look up toward your thumbs. Stretch up from your hips as you arch slightly at the top of your back. Make this intentionally exploratory without forcing anything. Take 3 full breaths (15 seconds).

3. **Mountain Pose:** Stand tall, inhale, and reach your arms straight up to the ceiling. Ground down through the soles of your feet and squeeze your inner thighs together. Keep your lower ribs in and turn your pinkies in-ward to relax your shoulders away from your ears. Take 10 full breaths (1 minute). Return your arms to your sides.

4. **Standing Forward Bend:** Exhale and hinge at your hips. Let your torso drape over your thighs as you reach your fingers toward the ground, bending as far as you can comfortably to release your lower back. Take 5 full breaths (30 seconds).

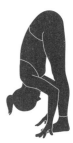

Focus Sequence 3

1. **Mountain Pose:** Stand tall, inhale, and reach your arms straight up. Ground through the soles of your feet and squeeze your inner thighs together. Keep your lower ribs in and turn your pinkies inward to relax your shoulders away from your ears. Take 5 full breaths (30 seconds). Return your arms to your sides.

2. **Tree Pose I:** Sink your weight into your left leg and draw the sole of your right foot up to the inside of your left leg. Place your foot either on your calf or your inner thigh, avoiding your knee, and splay your knee out to the side. Draw your palms to prayer at your heart center. Take 5 full breaths (30 seconds). Repeat Tree Pose I on the other side.

3. **Mountain Pose:** Stand tall, inhale, and reach your arms straight up. Ground through the soles of your feet and squeeze your inner thighs together. Keep your lower ribs in and turn your pinkies inward to relax your shoulders away from your ears. Take 3 full breaths (15 seconds). Return your arms to your sides.

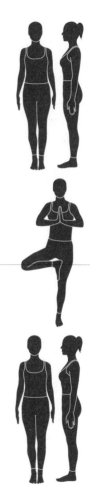

4. **Standing Forward Bend:** Exhale and hinge at your hips. Let your torso drape over your thighs as you reach your fingers toward the ground, bending as far as you can comfortably to release your lower back.

5. **Standing Half-Forward Bend:** For one breath in, place your hands on the chair in front of you and breathe. Create one line of energy from your tailbone to the top of your head. Plug your shoulders into their sockets and engage your shoulder blades together and down your back.

6. **Supported Legs Up the Wall:** Lie down on your back facing a wall and bring your knees into your chest, positioning your buttocks close to the wall. Lift your hips and place your elbows on the ground (place folded blankets or bolsters under your lower back and hips, if you prefer). Straighten your legs and send your feet straight up to the ceiling, using the wall as support. Raise your arms to the sides of your head with your elbows bent and your palms up. Take 10 full breaths (1 minute).

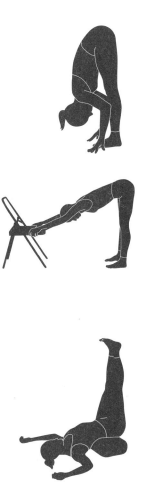

7. **Basic Relaxation Pose:** Extend your arms and legs flat on your mat. With your palms facing up, surrender to all effort and allow your body to melt into your mat. Let your muscles relax completely and allow all tension to drip off your fingertips and toes. Relax and breathe for 1 minute.

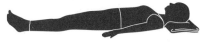

Focus Sequence 4

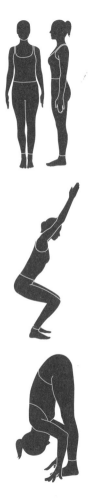

1. **Mountain Pose:** Stand tall, inhale, and reach your arms straight up to the ceiling. Ground down through the soles of your feet and squeeze your inner thighs together. Keep your lower ribs in and turn your pinkies inward to relax your shoulders away from your ears. Take 10 full breaths (1 minute). Return your arms to your sides.

2. **Chair Pose:** Inhale, bend your knees, and sweep your arms up toward the ceiling. Sink your weight into your hips and let the weight sink all the way down into your heels. Squeeze your inner thighs together, keep your lower ribs in, and relax your shoulders away from your ears. Take 5 full breaths (30 seconds).

3. **Standing Forward Bend:** Exhale and hinge at your hips. Let your torso drape over your thighs as you reach your fingers toward the ground, bending as far as you can comfortably to release your lower back. Take 3 full breaths (15 seconds).

4. **Downward-Facing Dog:** Exhale, plant your hands, and step your feet back behind you. Send your hips up high and fold your torso toward your thighs. Draw your thighs away from your kneecaps by engaging your quadriceps. Sink your heels toward the mat. Take 10 full breaths (1 minute).

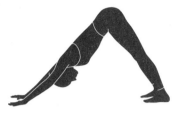

Focus Sequence 5

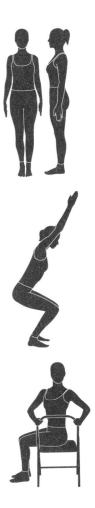

1. **Mountain Pose:** Stand tall, inhale, and reach your arms straight up. Ground through the soles of your feet and squeeze your inner thighs together. Keep your lower ribs in and turn your pinkies inward to relax your shoulders away from your ears. Take 10 full breaths (1 minute). Return your arms to your sides.

2. **Chair Pose:** Inhale, bend your knees, and sweep your arms up toward the ceiling. Sink your weight into your hips and let the weight sink all the way down into your heels. Squeeze your inner thighs together, keep your lower ribs in, and relax your shoulders away from your ears. Take 5 full breaths (30 seconds).

3. **Chair Twist:** Sit down sideways on a chair. Exhale and bring your palms to prayer at your heart center. Twist your torso toward the back of the chair, bringing your right elbow to the outside of your right thigh and grasping the back of the chair. Grasp the other side of the chair back with your other hand. Use your arms as leverage to peel your torso away from your thighs and twist open even more. Take 5 full breaths (30 seconds). Repeat Chair Twist on the other side.

Focus Sequence 6

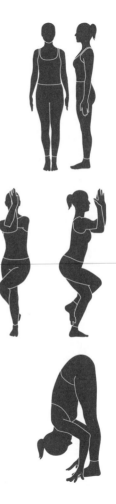

1. **Mountain Pose:** Stand tall, inhale, and reach your arms straight up. Ground through the soles of your feet and squeeze your inner thighs together. Keep your lower ribs in and turn your pinkies inward to relax your shoulders away from your ears. Take 10 full breaths (1 minute). Return your arms to your sides.

2. **Eagle Pose:** Wrap your right arm under your left arm and bring your palms together. Bring your elbows in line with your shoulders. Wrap your left leg over your right and either wrap your foot all the way around your calf or use your foot as a kickstand. Squeeze everything in toward the midline of your body. Take 5 full breaths (30 seconds). Repeat on the other side.

3. **Standing Forward Bend:** Exhale and hinge at your hips. Let your torso drape over your thighs and reach your fingers toward the ground, bending as far as you can comfortably to release your lower back. Take 5 full breaths (30 seconds).

Focus Sequence 7

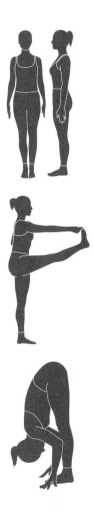

1. **Mountain Pose:** Stand tall, inhale, and reach your arms straight up. Ground through the soles of your feet and squeeze your inner thighs together. Keep your lower ribs in and turn your pinkies inward to relax your shoulders away from your ears. Take 10 full breaths (1 minute). Return your arms to your sides.

2. **Extended Hand on the Foot Pose:** Shift your weight onto your left leg and draw your right knee up toward your chest. Grab your big toe with your right hand, using your index and middle fingers. Straighten your leg out in front of you as far as comfortably possible, keeping your shoulders directly over your hips and your chest open. Take 5 full breaths (30 seconds). Repeat Extended Hand on the Foot Pose on the other side.

3. **Standing Forward Bend:** Exhale and hinge at your hips. Let your torso drape over your thighs and reach your fingers toward the ground, bending as far as you can comfortably to release your lower back. Take 5 full breaths (30 seconds).

Focus Sequence 8

1. **Mountain Pose:** Stand tall, inhale, and reach your arms straight up. Ground through the soles of your feet and squeeze your inner thighs together. Keep your lower ribs in and turn your pinkies inward to relax your shoulders away from your ears. Take 10 full breaths (1 minute). Return your arms to your sides.

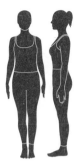

2. **Standing Forward Bend:** Exhale and hinge at your hips. Let your torso drape over your thighs and reach your fingers toward the ground, bending as far as you can comfortably to release your lower back. Take 3 full breaths (15 seconds).

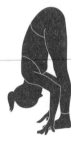

3. **Standing Half-Forward Bend:** For one breath in, place your hands on the chair in front of you and breathe. Create one line of energy from your tailbone to the top of your head. Plug your shoulders into their sockets and engage your shoulder blades together and down your back.

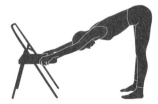

4. **Extended Side Angle Pose:** Inhale, then exhale and move one foot between your hands. Ground your back heel down, bend into your front knee, and twist from your lower torso as you reach your left hand up toward the ceiling. Keep your right hand on the floor next to your foot. Work to stack your shoulders on top of each other and spiral your ribs toward the ceiling. Reach up toward your top hand rather than down toward the ground. Take 5 full breaths (30 seconds). Repeat Extended Side Angle Pose on the other side.

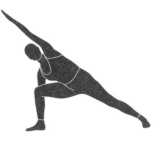

5. **Standing Forward Bend:** Exhale and hinge at your hips. Let your torso drape over your thighs and reach your fingers toward the ground, bending as far as you can comfortably to release your lower back. Take 3 full breaths (15 seconds).

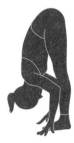

Focus Sequence 9

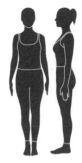

1. **Mountain Pose:** Stand tall, inhale, and reach your arms straight up. Ground through the soles of your feet and squeeze your inner thighs together. Keep your lower ribs in and turn your pinkies inward to relax your shoulders away from your ears. Take 10 full breaths (1 minute). Return your arms to your sides.

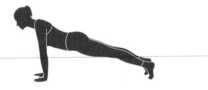

2. **Plank Pose:** Exhale, plant your hands palms down, shoulder-width apart, and extend your legs behind you. Place your feet hip-width apart with your toes pointed down. Create one long line of energy from your heels to the top of your head. Take 3 full breaths (15 seconds).

3. **Cobra Pose:** Exhale, lower down to your belly, bring your hands directly underneath your shoulders by your lower ribs, and bring your legs together. On an inhale, peel your chest away from the mat using your body and putting little to no weight on your hands. Straighten out your legs and stretch your chest forward with your hands palms down, arms lightly bent at the elbow, and

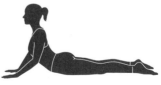

your chest and head aligned. Take 3 full
breaths (15 seconds).

4. **Locust Pose:** Extend your arms
above your head with your palms
facing each other. Inhale and lift
your arms, legs, and chest off your
mat; as you exhale, roll onto the
soft part of your belly. Squeeze
your inner thighs together and
keep your gaze down to protect your
neck. Engage your muscles to lift
as high as you can while continuing
to breathe. Take 3 full breaths (15
seconds).

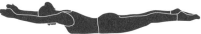

5. **Plank Pose:** Exhale, plant your hands
palms down, shoulder-width apart, and
extend your legs behind you. Place
your feet hip-width apart with your
toes pointed down. Create one long
line of energy from your heels to the
top of your head. Take 3 full breaths (15
seconds).

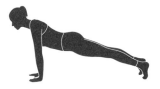

6. **Downward-Facing Dog:** Exhale, plant your hands, and step your feet back behind you. Send your hips up high and fold your torso toward your thighs. Draw your thighs away from your kneecaps by engaging your quadriceps. Sink your heels toward the mat. Take 10 full breaths (1 minute).

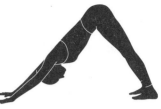

Focus Sequence 10

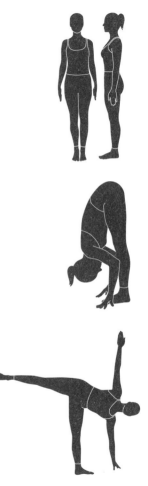

1. **Mountain Pose:** Stand tall, inhale, and reach your arms straight up to the ceiling. Ground down through the soles of your feet and squeeze your inner thighs together. Keep your lower ribs in and turn your pinkies inward to relax your shoulders away from your ears. Take 10 full breaths (1 minute). Return your arms to your sides.
2. **Standing Forward Bend:** Exhale and hinge at your hips. Let your torso drape over your thighs and reach your fingers toward the ground, bending as far as you can comfortably to release your lower back. Take 3 full breaths (15 seconds).
3. **Half-Moon Pose:** Inhale, send your right leg straight up behind you, and bring it parallel with the floor. Twist your torso open to the left and work to stack your shoulders directly over each other. Send your left arm down to the floor and your right arm up toward the ceiling. Take 5 full breaths (30 seconds). Repeat Half-Moon Pose on the other side.

4. **Warrior II:** Inhale as you move into Warrior II—ground your back heel down and move your hips to open along with your chest. Lower your arms to extend outward from your shoulders to your fingertips. Bend into your front knee up to 90 degrees and make sure it's stacked directly over your ankle. Keep your back leg engaged and externally rotate your front thigh. Take 5 full breaths (30 seconds). Repeat Warrior II on the other side.

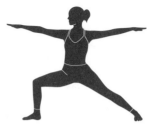

5. **Plank Pose:** Exhale, plant your hands palms down, shoulder-width apart, and extend your legs behind you. Place your feet hip-width apart with your toes pointed down. Create one long line of energy from your heels to the top of your head. Take 3 full breaths (15 seconds).

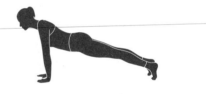

6. **Standing Forward Bend:** Exhale and hinge at your hips. Let your torso drape over your thighs and reach your fingers toward the ground, bending as far as you can comfortably to release your lower back. Take 3 full breaths (15 seconds).

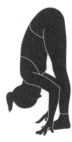

YOGA SEQUENCES FOR BALANCE

Much of yoga focuses on balance, both in terms of muscle use and in an ability to balance the needs of your mind and body. Even simple asanas like Mountain Pose teach you to find symmetry and balance in your body. Let these sequences bring mental and physical stability to your day.

Balance Sequence 1

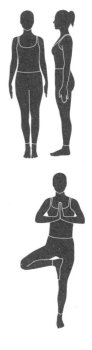

1. **Mountain Pose:** Stand tall, inhale, and reach your arms straight up to the ceiling. Ground down through the soles of your feet and squeeze your inner thighs together. Keep your lower ribs in and turn your pinkies inward to relax your shoulders away from your ears. Take 10 full breaths (1 minute). Return your arms to your sides.

2. **Tree Pose I:** Sink your weight into your left leg and draw the sole of your right foot up to the inside of your left leg. Place your foot either on your calf or your inner thigh, avoiding your knee, and splay your knee out to the side. Draw your palms to prayer at your heart center. Take 5 full breaths (30 seconds). Repeat on the other side.

3. **Mountain Pose:** Stand tall, inhale, and reach your arms straight up to the ceiling. Ground down through the soles of your feet and squeeze your inner thighs together. Keep your lower ribs in and turn your pinkies inward to relax your shoulders away from your ears. Take 10 full breaths (1 minute). Return your arms to your sides.

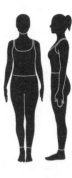

4. **Standing Forward Bend:** Exhale and hinge at your hips. Let your torso drape over your thighs and reach your fingers toward the ground, bending as far as you can comfortably to release your lower back. Take 3 full breaths (15 seconds).

5. **Downward-Facing Dog:** Exhale, plant your hands, and step your feet back behind you. Send your hips up high and fold your torso toward your thighs. Draw your thighs away from your kneecaps by engaging your quadriceps. Sink your heels toward the mat. Take 5 full breaths (30 seconds).

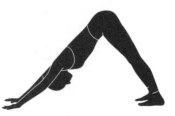

Balance Sequence 2

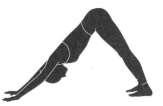

1. **Downward-Facing Dog:** Exhale, plant your hands, and step your feet back behind you. Send your hips up high and fold your torso toward your thighs. Draw your thighs away from your kneecaps by engaging your quadriceps. Sink your heels toward the mat. Take 5 full breaths (30 seconds).

2. **Standing Forward Bend:** Exhale and hinge at your hips. Let your torso drape over your thighs and reach your fingers toward the ground, bending as far as you can comfortably to release your lower back. Take 3 full breaths (15 seconds).

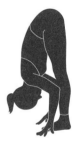

3. **Mountain Pose:** Stand tall, inhale, and reach your arms straight up to the ceiling. Ground down through the soles of your feet and squeeze your inner thighs together. Keep your lower ribs in and turn your pinkies inward to relax your shoulders away from your ears. Take 5 full breaths (30 seconds). Return your arms to your sides.

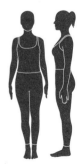

4. **Tree Pose I:** Sink your weight into your left leg and draw the sole of your right foot up to the inside of your left leg. Place your foot either on your calf or your inner thigh, avoiding your knee, and splay your knee out to the side. Draw your palms to prayer at your heart center. Take 5 full breaths (30 seconds). Repeat Tree Pose I on the other side.

5. **Mountain Pose:** Stand tall, inhale, and reach your arms straight up to the ceiling. Ground down through the soles of your feet and squeeze your inner thighs together. Keep your lower ribs in and turn your pinkies inward to relax your shoulders away from your ears. Take 3 full breaths (15 seconds). Return your arms to your sides.

6. **Standing Forward Bend:** Exhale and hinge at your hips. Let your torso drape over your thighs and reach your fingers toward the ground, bending as far as you can comfortably to release your lower back. Take 3 full breaths (15 seconds).

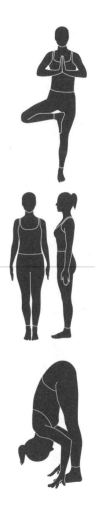

7. **Plank Pose:** Exhale, plant your hands palms down, shoulder-width apart, and extend your legs behind you. Place your feet hip-width apart with your toes pointed down. Create one long line of energy from your heels to the top of your head. Take 3 full breaths (15 seconds).

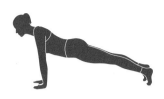

Balance Sequence 3

1. **Downward-Facing Dog:** Exhale, plant your hands, and step your feet back behind you. Send your hips up high and fold your torso toward your thighs. Draw your thighs away from your kneecaps by engaging your quadriceps. Sink your heels toward the mat. Take 5 full breaths (30 seconds).

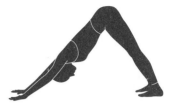

2. **Standing Forward Bend:** Exhale and hinge at your hips. Let your torso drape over your thighs and reach your fingers toward the ground, bending as far as you can comfortably to release your lower back. Take 3 full breaths (15 seconds).

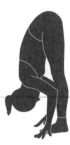

3. **Mountain Pose:** Stand tall, inhale, and reach your arms straight up to the ceiling. Ground down through the soles of your feet and squeeze your inner thighs together. Keep your lower ribs in and turn your pinkies inward to relax your shoulders away from your ears. Take 5 full breaths (30 seconds). Return your arms to your sides.

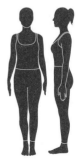

4. **Tree Pose II:** Sink your weight into your left/right standing leg. Draw the sole of your right/left foot to the inside of your left/right leg. Place your foot either on your calf or your inner thigh, avoiding your knee. Splay your knee out to the side and send your arms straight up toward the ceiling. Take 5 full breaths (30 seconds). Repeat Tree Pose II on the other side.

5. **Mountain Pose:** Stand tall, inhale, and reach your arms straight up to the ceiling. Ground down through the soles of your feet and squeeze your inner thighs together. Keep your lower ribs in and turn your pinkies inward to relax your shoulders away from your ears. Take 3 full breaths (15 seconds). Return your arms to your sides.

6. **Standing Forward Bend:** Exhale and hinge at your hips. Let your torso drape over your thighs and reach your fingers toward the ground, bending as far as you can comfortably to release your lower back. Take 3 full breaths (15 seconds).

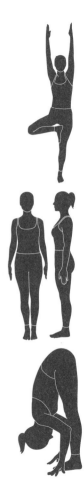

7. **Plank Pose:** Exhale, plant your hands palms down, shoulder-width apart, and extend your legs behind you. Place your feet hip-width apart with your toes pointed down. Create one long line of energy from your heels to the top of your head. Take 3 full breaths (15 seconds).

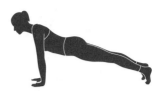

Balance Sequence 4

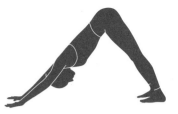

1. **Downward-Facing Dog:** Exhale, plant your hands, and step your feet back behind you. Send your hips up high and fold your torso toward your thighs. Draw your thighs away from your kneecaps by engaging your quadriceps. Sink your heels toward the mat. Take 5 full breaths (30 seconds).

2. **Standing Forward Bend:** Exhale and hinge at your hips. Let your torso drape over your thighs and reach your fingers toward the ground, bending as far as you can comfortably to release your lower back. Take 3 full breaths (15 seconds).

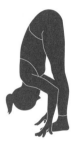

3. **Mountain Pose:** Stand tall, inhale, and reach your arms straight up to the ceiling. Ground down through the soles of your feet and squeeze your inner thighs together. Keep your lower ribs in and turn your pinkies inward to relax your shoulders away from your ears. Take 5 full breaths (30 seconds). Return your arms to your sides.

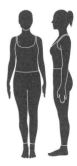

4. **Tree Pose I:** Sink your weight into your left leg and draw the sole of your right foot up to the inside of your left leg. Place your foot either on your calf or your inner thigh, avoiding your knee, and splay your knee out to the side. Draw your palms to prayer at your heart center. Take 5 full breaths (30 seconds). Repeat Tree Pose I on the other side.

5. **Tree Pose II:** Sink your weight into your left/right standing leg. Draw the sole of your right/left foot to the inside of your left/right leg. Place your foot either on your calf or your inner thigh, avoiding your knee. Splay your knee out to the side and send your arms straight up toward the ceiling. Take 5 full breaths (30 seconds). Repeat Tree Pose II on the other side.

6. **Mountain Pose:** Stand tall, inhale, and reach your arms straight up. Ground through the soles of your feet and squeeze your inner thighs together. Keep your lower ribs in and turn your pinkies inward to relax your shoulders away from your ears. Take 3 full breaths (15 seconds). Return your arms to your sides.

7. **Standing Forward Bend:** Exhale and hinge at your hips. Let your torso drape over your thighs and reach your fingers toward the ground, bending as far as you can comfortably to release your lower back. Take 3 full breaths (15 seconds).

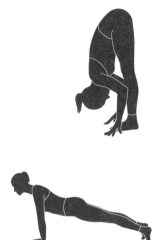

8. **Plank Pose:** Exhale, plant your hands palms down, shoulder-width apart, and extend your legs behind you. Place your feet hip-width apart with your toes pointed down. Create one long line of energy from your heels to the top of your head. Take 3 full breaths (15 seconds).

Balance Sequence 5

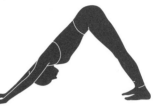

1. **Downward-Facing Dog:** Exhale, plant your hands, and step your feet back behind you. Send your hips up high and fold your torso toward your thighs. Draw your thighs away from your kneecaps by engaging your quadriceps. Sink your heels toward the mat. Take 5 full breaths (30 seconds).

2. **Standing Forward Bend:** Inhale and hinge at your hips. Let your torso drape over your thighs and reach your fingers toward the ground, bending as far as you can comfortably to release your lower back. Take 3 full breaths (15 seconds).

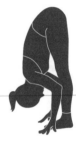

3. **Mountain Pose:** Stand tall, inhale, and reach your arms straight up to the ceiling. Ground down through the soles of your feet and squeeze your inner thighs together. Keep your lower ribs in and turn your pinkies inward to relax your shoulders away from your ears. Take 3 full breaths (15 seconds). Return your arms to your sides.

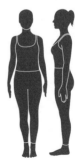

4. **Eagle Pose:** Wrap your right arm under your left arm and bring your palms together. Bring your elbows in line with your shoulders. Wrap your left leg over your right and either wrap your foot all the way around your calf or use your foot as a kickstand. Squeeze everything in toward the midline of your body. Take 5 full breaths (30 seconds). Repeat Eagle Pose on the other side.

5. **Mountain Pose:** Stand tall, inhale, and reach your arms straight up to the ceiling. Ground down through the soles of your feet and squeeze your inner thighs together. Keep your lower ribs in and turn your pinkies inward to relax your shoulders away from your ears. Take 3 full breaths (15 seconds). Return your arms to your sides.

6. **Standing Forward Bend:** Exhale and hinge at your hips. Let your torso drape over your thighs and reach your fingers toward the ground, bending as far as you can comfortably to release your lower back. Take 3 full breaths (15 seconds).

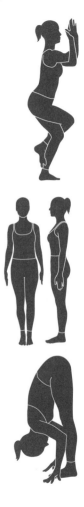

7. **Plank Pose:** Exhale, plant your hands palms down, shoulder-width apart, and extend your legs behind you. Place your feet hip-width apart with your toes pointed down. Create one long line of energy from your heels to the top of your head. Take 3 full breaths (15 seconds).

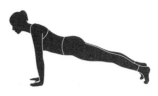

8. **Downward-Facing Dog:** Exhale, plant your hands, and step your feet back behind you. Send your hips up high and fold your torso toward your thighs. Draw your thighs away from your kneecaps by engaging your quadriceps. Sink your heels toward the mat. Take 5 full breaths (30 seconds).

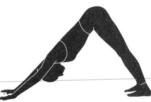

Balance Sequence 6

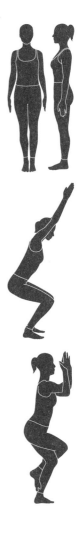

1. **Mountain Pose:** Stand tall, inhale, and reach your arms straight up. Ground through the soles of your feet and squeeze your inner thighs together. Keep your lower ribs in and turn your pinkies inward to relax your shoulders away from your ears. Take 5 full breaths (30 seconds). Return your arms to your sides.

2. **Chair Pose:** Inhale, bend your knees, and sweep your arms up toward the ceiling. Sink your weight into your hips and let the weight sink all the way down into your heels. Squeeze your inner thighs together, keep your lower ribs in, and relax your shoulders away from your ears. Take 5 full breaths (30 seconds).

3. **Eagle Pose:** Wrap your right arm under your left arm and bring your palms together. Bring your elbows in line with your shoulders. Wrap your left leg over your right and either wrap your foot all the way around your calf or use your foot as a kickstand. Squeeze everything in toward the midline of your body. Take 5 full breaths (30 seconds). Repeat Eagle Pose on the other side.

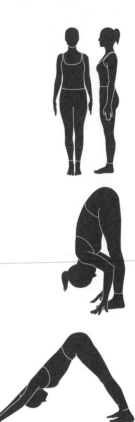

4. **Mountain Pose:** Stand tall, inhale, and reach your arms straight up to the ceiling. Ground down through the soles of your feet and squeeze your inner thighs together. Keep your lower ribs in and turn your pinkies inward to relax your shoulders away from your ears. Take 5 full breaths (30 seconds). Return your arms to your sides.

5. **Standing Forward Bend:** Exhale and hinge at your hips. Let your torso drape over your thighs and reach your fingers toward the ground, bending as far as you can comfortably to release your lower back. Take 3 full breaths (15 seconds).

6. **Downward-Facing Dog:** Exhale, plant your hands, and step your feet back behind you. Send your hips up high and fold your torso toward your thighs. Draw your thighs away from your kneecaps by engaging your quadriceps. Sink your heels toward the mat. Take 5 full breaths (30 seconds).

Balance Sequence 7

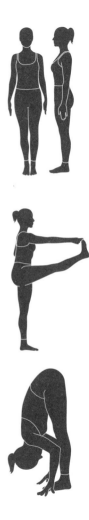

1. **Mountain Pose:** Stand tall, inhale, and reach your arms straight up. Ground through the soles of your feet and squeeze your inner thighs together. Keep your lower ribs in and turn your pinkies inward to relax your shoulders away from your ears. Take 5 full breaths (30 seconds). Return your arms to your sides.

2. **Extended Hand on the Foot Pose:** Shift your weight onto your left leg and draw your right knee up toward your chest. Grab your big toe with your right hand, using your index and middle fingers. Straighten your leg out in front of you as far as comfortably possible, keeping your shoulders directly over your hips and your chest open. Take 5 full breaths (30 seconds). Repeat Extended Hand on the Foot Pose on the other side.

3. **Standing Forward Bend:** Exhale and hinge at your hips. Let your torso drape over your thighs and reach your fingers toward the ground, bending as far as you can comfortably to release your lower back. Take 3 full breaths (15 seconds).

4. **Downward-Facing Dog:** Exhale, plant your hands, and step your feet back behind you. Send your hips up high and fold your torso toward your thighs. Draw your thighs away from your kneecaps by engaging your quadriceps. Sink your heels toward the mat. Take 10 full breaths (1 minute).

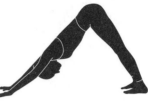

Balance Sequence 8

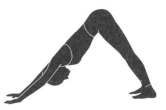

1. **Downward-Facing Dog:** Exhale, plant your hands, and step your feet back behind you. Send your hips up high and fold your torso toward your thighs. Draw your thighs away from your kneecaps by engaging your quadriceps. Sink your heels toward the mat. Take 5 full breaths (30 seconds).

2. **Standing Forward Bend:** Exhale and hinge at your hips. Let your torso drape over your thighs and reach your fingers toward the ground, bending as far as you can comfortably to release your lower back. Take 3 full breaths (15 seconds).

3. **Mountain Pose:** Stand tall, inhale, and reach your arms straight up to the ceiling. Ground down through the soles of your feet and squeeze your inner thighs together. Keep your lower ribs in and turn your pinkies inward to relax your shoulders away from your ears. Take 5 full breaths (30 seconds). Return your arms to your sides.

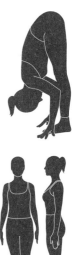

4. **Extended Hand on the Foot Pose:** Shift your weight onto your left leg and draw your right knee up toward your chest. Grab your big toe with your right hand, using your index and middle fingers. Straighten your leg out in front of you as far as comfortably possible, keeping your shoulders directly over your hips and your chest open. Take 5 full breaths (30 seconds). Repeat Extended Hand on the Foot Pose on the other side.

5. **Mountain Pose:** Stand tall, inhale, and reach your arms straight up. Ground through the soles of your feet and squeeze your inner thighs together. Keep your lower ribs in and turn your pinkies inward to relax your shoulders away from your ears. Take 3 full breaths (15 seconds). Return your arms to your sides.

6. **Standing Forward Bend:** Exhale and hinge at your hips. Let your torso drape over your thighs and reach your fingers toward the ground, bending as far as you can comfortably to release your lower back. Inhale.

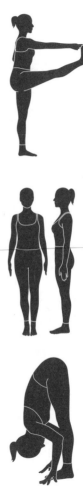

7. **Plank Pose:** Exhale, plant your hands palms down, shoulder-width apart, and extend your legs behind you. Place your feet hip-width apart with your toes pointed down. Create one long line of energy from your heels to the top of your head. Take 3 full breaths (15 seconds).

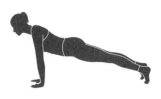

Balance Sequence 9

1. **Downward-Facing Dog:** Exhale, plant your hands, and step your feet back behind you. Send your hips up high and fold your torso toward your thighs. Draw your thighs away from your kneecaps by engaging your quadriceps. Sink your heels toward the mat. Take 3 full breaths (15 seconds).

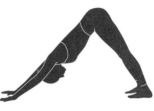

2. **Standing Forward Bend:** Exhale and hinge at your hips. Let your torso drape over your thighs and reach your fingers toward the ground, bending as far as you can comfortably to release your lower back. Take 3 full breaths (15 seconds).

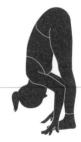

3. **Warrior II:** Inhale as you move into Warrior II— ground your back heel down and move your hips to open along with your chest. Lower your arms to extend outward from your shoulders to your fingertips. Bend into your front knee up to 90 degrees and make sure it's stacked directly over your ankle. Keep your back leg engaged and externally rotate your front thigh. Take 5 full breaths (30 seconds). Repeat Warrior II on the other side.

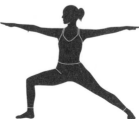

4. **Half-Moon Pose:** Inhale, send your right leg straight up behind you, and bring it parallel with the floor. Twist your torso open to the left and work to stack your shoulders directly over each other. Send your left arm down to the floor and your right arm up toward the ceiling. Take 5 full breaths (30 seconds). Repeat Half-Moon Pose on the other side.

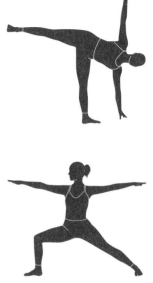

5. **Warrior II:** Inhale as you move into Warrior II—ground your back heel down and move your hips to open along with your chest. Lower your arms to extend outward from your shoulders to your fingertips. Bend into your front knee up to 90 degrees and make sure it's stacked directly over your ankle. Keep your back leg engaged and externally rotate your front thigh. Take 3 full breaths (15 seconds). Repeat Warrior II on the other side.

6. **Plank Pose:** Exhale, plant your hands palms down, shoulder-width apart, and extend your legs behind you. Place your feet hip-width apart with your toes pointed down. Create one long line of energy from your heels to the top of your head. Inhale.

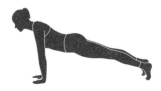

7. **Downward-Facing Dog:** Exhale, plant your hands, and step your feet back behind you. Send your hips up high and fold your torso toward your thighs. Draw your thighs away from your kneecaps by engaging your quadriceps. Sink your heels toward the mat. Take 3 full breaths (15 seconds).

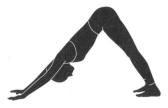

Balance Sequence 10

1. **Downward-Facing Dog:** Exhale, plant your hands, and step your feet back behind you. Send your hips up high and fold your torso toward your thighs. Draw your thighs away from your kneecaps by engaging your quadriceps. Sink your heels toward the mat. Take 3 full breaths (15 seconds).

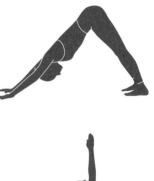

2. **Warrior I:** Inhale, then exhale and move one foot between your hands. Inhale into the position—ground your back heel down, bend your front knee into a 90-degree angle, stack your shoulders over your hips, and reach your arms straight up to the ceiling. Square your hips by drawing your front leg's outer hip back and pressing your opposite hip forward. Take 5 full breaths (30 seconds). Repeat Warrior I on the other side.

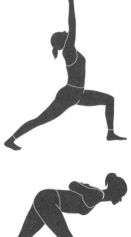

3. **Intense Side Stretch Pose:** Exhale, keep your feet where they are, and hinge at your hips, leaning down toward your front leg. Keep your back and neck straight and lead with your chest. Fold your arms behind your back. Take 5 full breaths (30 seconds).

Repeat Intense Side Stretch Pose on the other side.

4. **Warrior I:** Inhale, then exhale and move one foot between your hands. Inhale into the position—ground your back heel down, bend your front knee into a 90-degree angle, stack your shoulders over your hips, and reach your arms straight up to the ceiling. Square your hips by drawing your front leg's outer hip back and pressing your opposite hip forward. Take 5 full breaths (30 seconds). Repeat Warrior I on the other side.

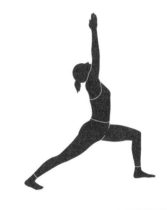

5. **Plank Pose:** Exhale, plant your hands palms down, shoulder-width apart, and extend your legs behind you. Place your feet hip-width apart with your toes pointed down. Create one long line of energy from your heels to the top of your head. Take 3 full breaths (15 seconds).

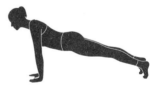

YOGA SEQUENCES FOR PEACE

The world around us is a busy, noisy place. Try to take a few moments during the day to allow your body and mind to find stillness. Do your best to find a quiet spot for these sequences, whether it's in a room or office with the door closed or in an empty meadow. You'll find that you begin to relish your yoga practice as a reliable place to enjoy quiet, mindful reflection.

Peace Sequence 1

1. **Child's Pose:** Exhale, kneel down on your mat, and bring your big toes together behind you. Spread out your knees and rest your torso on your thighs. Extend your arms above your head and rest your forehead on the mat. Spread your fingers evenly and wide. With every inhale, reach your fingertips toward the front of the mat and with every exhale, sink your hips closer to your heels. Take 20 full breaths (2 minutes).

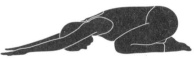

2. **Cat-Cow:** Exhale and drop down to your hands and knees. Inhale, drop your belly, and arch your back, raising your tailbone. Lift your gaze as you find expansion across your chest. Exhale, arch your spine up, and lower your tailbone. Let your head hang heavy and look down between your thighs. Take 10 full breaths (1 minute).

3. **Basic Relaxation Pose:** Lie flat on your mat and extend your arms and legs. With your palms facing up, surrender to all effort and allow your body to melt into your mat. Let your muscles relax completely and allow all tension to drip off your fingertips and toes. Relax and breathe for 2 minutes.

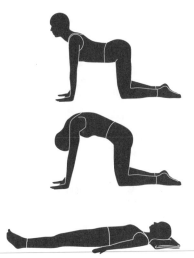

Peace Sequence 2

1. **Child's Pose:** Exhale, kneel down on your mat, and bring your big toes together behind you. Spread out your knees and rest your torso on your thighs. Extend your arms above your head and rest your forehead on the mat. Spread your fingers evenly and wide. With every inhale, reach your fingertips toward the front of the mat and with every exhale, sink your hips closer to your heels. Take 10 full breaths (1 minute).

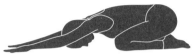

2. **Head-to-Knee Pose:** Sit on your mat and extend your legs in front of you. Draw the sole of your right foot to your inner left thigh and extend your left leg in front of you. Reach your arms forward and fold over your extended leg, keeping your back flat. Take 10 full breaths (1 minute). Repeat Head-to-Knee Pose on the other side.

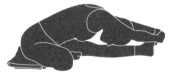

3. **Basic Relaxation Pose:** Lie flat on your mat and extend your arms and legs. With your palms facing up, surrender to all effort and allow your body to melt into your mat. Let your muscles relax completely and allow all tension to drip off your fingertips and toes. Relax and breathe for 2 minutes.

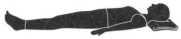

Peace Sequence 3

1. **Child's Pose:** Exhale, kneel down on your mat, and bring your big toes together behind you. Spread out your knees and rest your torso on your thighs. Extend your arms above your head and rest your forehead on the mat. Spread your fingers evenly and wide. With every inhale, reach your fingertips toward the front of the mat and with every exhale, sink your hips closer to your heels. Take 10 full breaths (1 minute).

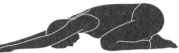

2. **Pigeon Pose:** Bring your right leg in front of you, bent at the knee, and extend your left leg straight behind you with the top of your foot flat on your mat. Square your hips the best you can and then draw your chest forward as you walk your hands out in front of you, keeping your back straight. Take 10 full breaths (1 minute). Repeat Pigeon Pose on the other side.

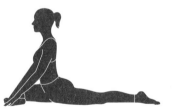

3. **Basic Relaxation Pose:** Lie flat on your mat and extend your arms and legs. With your palms facing up, surrender to all effort and allow your body to melt into your mat. Let your muscles relax completely and allow all tension to drip off your fingertips and toes. Relax and breathe for 2 minutes.

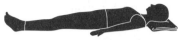

Peace Sequence 4

1. **Child's Pose:** Exhale, kneel down on your mat, and bring your big toes together behind you. Spread out your knees and rest your torso on your thighs. Extend your arms above your head and rest your forehead on the mat. Spread your fingers evenly and wide. With every inhale, reach your fingertips toward the front of the mat and with every exhale, sink your hips closer to your heels. Take 10 full breaths (1 minute).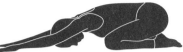

2. **Easy Pose:** Sit up tall on one or two folded blankets with your legs crossed. Rest your hands on the mat beside your hips or bring your palms to prayer at your heart center and close your eyes. Take 20 full breaths (2 minutes).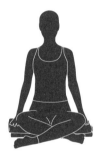

3. **Basic Relaxation Pose:** Lie flat on your mat and extend your arms and legs. With your palms facing up, surrender to all effort and allow your body to melt into your mat. Let your muscles relax completely and allow all tension to drip off your fingertips and toes. Relax and breathe for 2 minutes.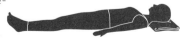

Peace Sequence 5

1. **Child's Pose:** Exhale, kneel down on your mat, and bring your big toes together behind you. Spread out your knees and rest your torso on your thighs. Extend your arms above your head and rest your forehead on the mat. Spread your fingers evenly and wide. With every inhale, reach your fingertips toward the front of the mat and with every exhale, sink your hips closer to your heels. Take 10 full breaths (1 minute).

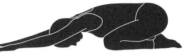

2. **Reclining Hand-to-Big-Toe Pose I:** Lie on your back and bring your knees into your chest. Grab your right big toe with your index and middle finger (or wrap a strap around the ball of your foot) and straighten out your leg in front of you as far as you can. Extend your left leg and keep your shoulders and head flat on the mat. Take 10 full breaths (1 minute). Repeat Reclining Hand-to-Big-Toe Pose I on the other side.

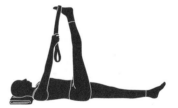

3. **Basic Relaxation Pose:** Extend your arms and legs flat on your mat. With your palms facing up, surrender to all effort and allow 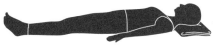 your body to melt into your mat. Let your muscles relax completely and allow all tension to drip off your fingertips and toes. Relax and breathe for 2 minutes.

Peace Sequence 6

1. **Child's Pose:** Exhale, kneel down on your mat, and bring your big toes together behind you. Spread out your knees and rest your torso on your thighs. Extend your arms above your head and rest your forehead on the mat. Spread your fingers evenly and wide. With every inhale, reach your fingertips toward the front of the mat and with every exhale, sink your hips closer to your heels. Take 10 full breaths (1 minute).

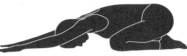

2. **Supported Legs Up the Wall Pose:** Lie down on your back facing a wall and bring your knees into your chest, positioning your buttocks close to the wall. Lift your hips and place your elbows on the ground (place folded blankets or bolsters under your lower back and hips, if you prefer). Straighten your legs and send your feet straight up to the ceiling, using the

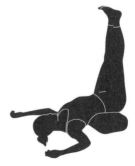

wall as support. Raise your arms to the sides of your head with your elbows bent and your palms up. Take 20 full breaths (2 minutes).

3. **Restorative Bridge Pose:** Put extra supports under your back. Lie down with your whole body and legs on the bolsters, so the bottom edge of your 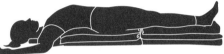 shoulder blades are on the upper edge of the top bolster. Loop a belt firmly around the middle of your thighs so they will not be able to roll apart. Relax and breathe for 2 minutes.

Peace Sequence 7

1. **Child's Pose:** Exhale, kneel down on your mat, and bring your big toes together behind you. Spread out your knees and rest your torso on your thighs. Extend your arms above your head and rest your forehead on the mat. Spread your fingers evenly and wide. With every inhale, reach your fingertips toward the front of the mat and with every exhale, sink your hips closer to your heels. Take 10 full breaths (1 minute).

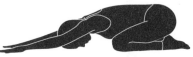

2. **Seated Straight-Leg Forward Bend:** Sit with your legs extended in front of you. Inhale to lengthen your spine, exhale, then hinge at your hips and reach for your toes, keeping your back flat. Clasp your hands together with your palms out, leaning forward as far as you can. Take 20 full breaths (2 minutes).

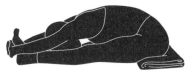

3. **Basic Relaxation Pose:** Lie flat on your mat and extend your arms and legs. With your palms facing up, surrender to all effort and allow your body to melt into your mat. Let your muscles relax completely and allow all tension to drip off your fingertips and toes. Relax and breathe for 2 minutes.

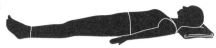

Peace Sequence 8

1. **Child's Pose:** Exhale, kneel down on your mat, and bring your big toes together behind you. Spread out your knees and rest your torso on your thighs. Extend your arms above your head and rest your forehead on the mat. Spread your fingers evenly and wide. With every inhale, reach your fingertips toward the front of the mat and with every exhale, sink your hips closer to your heels. Take 10 full breaths (1 minute).

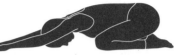

2. **Belly Twist:** Lie on your back and as you inhale, draw your knees into your chest. As you exhale, let your legs drop over to your left side, keeping your legs together and bent and your torso and arms flat on the mat. Twist your hips so your legs rest flat on the mat with your knees stacked on top of each other. Extend your arms out to the right and left in line with your shoulders and send your gaze over to the left for the full expression of this twist. Take 10 full breaths (1 minute). Repeat Belly Twist on the other side.

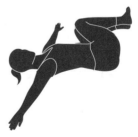

3. **Basic Relaxation Pose:** Extend your arms and legs flat on your mat. With your palms facing up, surrender to all effort and allow your body to melt into your mat. Let your muscles relax completely and allow all tension to drip off your fingertips and toes. Relax and breathe for 2 minutes.

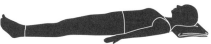

Peace Sequence 9

1. **Child's Pose:** Exhale, kneel down on your mat, and bring your big toes together behind you. Spread out your knees and rest your torso on your thighs. Extend your arms above your head and rest your forehead on the mat. Spread your fingers evenly and wide. With every inhale, reach your fingertips toward the front of the mat and with every exhale, sink your hips closer to your heels. Take 10 full breaths (1 minute).

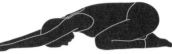

2. **Sage Twist:** Sit on your mat with your knees bent (place a folded blanket under your buttocks if it is more comfortable). Extend your left leg, place the fingertips of your right hand on the mat, and twist your torso to the right. Raise your left arm and press your elbow against the outside of your right upper thigh, near the knee, using this as leverage to twist your spine further and open your chest more. If you prefer, you can cross your right leg over the

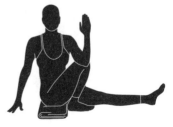

top of your left leg to enhance the twist. Take 10 full breaths (1 minute). Repeat Sage Twist on the other side.

3. **Basic Relaxation Pose:** Lie flat on your mat and extend your arms and legs. With your palms facing up, surrender to all effort and allow your body to melt into your mat. Let your muscles relax completely and allow all tension to drip off your fingertips and toes. Relax and breathe for 2 minutes.

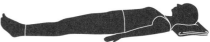

Peace Sequence 10

1. **Child's Pose:** Exhale, kneel down on your mat, and bring your big toes together behind you. Spread out your knees and rest your torso on your thighs. Extend your arms above your head and rest your forehead on the mat. Spread your fingers evenly and wide. With every inhale, reach your fingertips toward the front of the mat and with every exhale, sink your hips closer to your heels. Take 10 full breaths (1 minute).

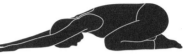

2. **Seated Wide-Angle Pose:** Sit on your mat and extend your legs in front of you. Spread your legs as far apart as is comfortable. Inhale and lengthen through your spine. As you exhale, crawl your fingers out in front of you, lowering yourself as far as you can while keeping your back straight. Grasp your legs or feet with your hands and look straight ahead as you relax into the pose. Take 20 full breaths (2 minutes).

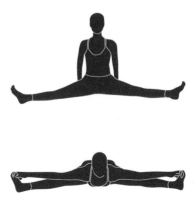

3. **Basic Relaxation Pose:** Lie flat on your mat and extend your arms and legs. With your palms facing up, surrender to all effort and allow your body to melt into your mat. Let your muscles relax completely and allow all tension to drip off your fingertips and toes. Relax and breathe for 2 minutes.

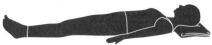

SEQUENCES
SPIRIT

YOGA SEQUENCES FOR RELAXATION

It can be difficult to truly relax—to fully let go of the day's responsibilities, worries, and to-do lists. Practicing yoga is a very effective way to encourage yourself to relax. You'll find yourself breathing fully and thinking about your posture and not about your next presentation at work.

Relaxation Sequence 1

1. **Bound Angle Pose:** Sit up tall on your mat. Bring the soles of your feet together in front of you and let your knees drop out to the sides. Hold your feet in your hands and pull them in toward your inner thighs as far as you can comfortably. Bring your arms in flat against your torso and place your fingertips on the mat behind your hips. Take 10 full breaths (1 minute).

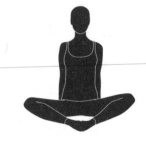

2. **Bridge Pose:** Lie down on your back, bend your knees, and place your feet a bit more than hip-width apart, flat on the mat. Inhale as you raise your hips. Exhale, shimmy your shoulders under-

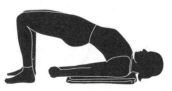

neath you, and extend your arms, clenching your hands into fists. Breathe air into your belly and find space across your chest. Take 20 full breaths (2 minutes).

3. **Basic Relaxation Pose:** Lie flat on your mat and extend your arms and legs. With your palms facing up, surrender to all effort and allow your body to melt into your mat. Let your muscles relax completely and allow all tension to drip off your fingertips and toes. Relax and breathe for 2 minutes.

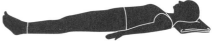

Relaxation Sequence 2

1. **Bound Angle Pose:** Sit up tall on your mat. Bring the soles of your feet together in front of you and let your knees drop out to the sides. Hold your feet in your hands and pull them in toward your inner thighs as far as you can comfortably. Bring your arms in flat against your torso and place your fingertips on the mat behind your hips. Take 10 full breaths (1 minute).

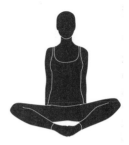

2. **Supported Bound Angle Pose:** Lie on your back and bend your knees (place folded blankets or bolsters under your head, back, and knees, if you prefer). Bring the soles of your feet together to touch and allow your knees to splay out to the sides. Close your eyes and extend your arms out to your sides as you breathe. Take 20 full breaths (2 minutes).

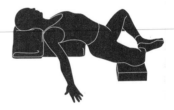

3. **Basic Relaxation Pose:** Extend your arms and legs flat on your mat. With your palms facing up, surrender to all effort and allow your body to melt into your mat. Let your muscles relax completely and allow all tension to drip off your fingertips and toes. Relax and breathe for 2 minutes.

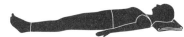

Relaxation Sequence 3

1. **Bound Angle Pose:** Sit up tall on your mat. Bring the soles of your feet together in front of you and let your knees drop out to the sides. Hold your feet in your hands and pull them in toward your inner thighs as far as you can comfortably. Bring your arms in flat against your torso and place your fingertips on the mat behind your hips. Take 10 full breaths (1 minute).

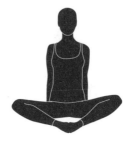

2. **Sideways Wide-Angle Pose:** Sit on your mat and extend your legs in front of you. Spread your legs as far apart as is comfortable. Inhale and lengthen through your spine. Place your right fingertips behind you and your left fingertips on the floor in front of your pubis. Press your fingertips down and ground your legs and buttocks as you inhale and lift your spine and the sides of your body. Exhale and gently rotate your body toward your right leg. Take 10 full breaths (1 minute). Repeat on the other side. Take 10 full breaths (1 minute).

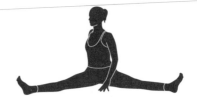

3. **Basic Relaxation Pose:** Lie flat on your 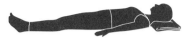 mat and extend your arms and legs. With your palms facing up, surrender to all effort and allow your body to melt into your mat. Let your muscles relax completely and allow all tension to drip off your fingertips and toes. Relax and breathe for 2 minutes.

Relaxation Sequence 4

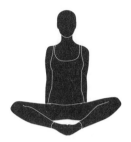

1. **Bound Angle Pose:** Sit up tall on your mat. Bring the soles of your feet together in front of you and let your knees drop out to the sides. Hold your feet in your hands and pull them in toward your inner thighs as far as you can comfortably. Bring your arms in flat against your torso and place your fingertips on the mat behind your hips. Take 10 full breaths (1 minute).

2. **Seated Straight-Leg Forward Bend:** Sit with your legs extended in front of you. Inhale to lengthen your spine, exhale, then hinge at your hips and reach for your toes, keeping your back flat. Clasp your hands together with your palms out, leaning forward as far as you can. Take 20 full breaths (2 minutes).

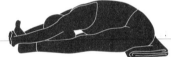

3. **Basic Relaxation Pose:** Lie flat on your mat and extend your arms and legs. With your palms facing up, surrender to all effort and allow your body to melt into your mat. Let your muscles relax completely and allow all tension to drip off your fingertips and toes. Relax and breathe for 2 minutes.

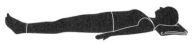

Relaxation Sequence 5

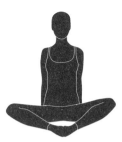

1. **Bound Angle Pose:** Sit up tall on your mat. Bring the soles of your feet together in front of you and let your knees drop out to the sides. Hold your feet in your hands and pull them in toward your inner thighs as far as you can comfortably. Bring your arms in flat against your torso and place your fingertips on the mat behind your hips. Take 10 full breaths (1 minute).

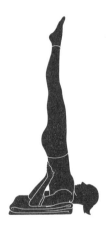

2. **Supported Shoulderstand:** Lie down on your back and bring your knees into your chest (place folded blankets or bolsters under your shoulders and arms, if you prefer). Lift your hips and place your elbows on the ground, bringing the base of your palms to your lower back and pushing yourself up onto your shoulders. Straighten your legs and send your toes straight up to the ceiling. Take 20 full breaths (2 minutes).

3. **Basic Relaxation Pose:** Extend your arms and legs flat on your mat. With your palms facing up, surrender to all effort and allow your body to melt into your mat. Let your muscles relax completely and allow all tension to drip off your fingertips and toes. Relax and breathe for 2 minutes.

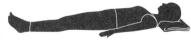

Relaxation Sequence 6

1. **Bound Angle Pose:** Sit up tall on your mat. Bring the soles of your feet together in front of you and let your knees drop out to the sides. Hold your feet in your hands and pull them in toward your inner thighs as far as you can comfortably. Bring your arms in flat against your torso and place your fingertips on the mat behind your hips. Take 10 full breaths (1 minute).

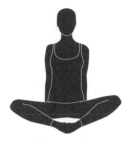

2. **Supported Legs Up the Wall:** Lie down on your back facing a wall and bring your knees into your chest, positioning your buttocks close to the wall. Lift your hips and place your elbows on the ground (place folded blankets or bolsters under your lower back and hips, if you prefer). Straighten your legs and send your feet straight up to the ceiling, using the wall as support. Raise your arms to the sides of your head with your elbows bent and your palms up. Take 20 full breaths (2 minutes).

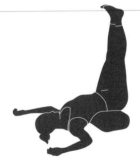

3. **Basic Relaxation Pose:** Extend your 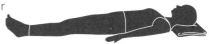 arms and legs flat on your mat. With your palms facing up, surrender to all effort and allow your body to melt into your mat. Let your muscles relax completely and allow all tension to drip off your fingertips and toes. Relax and breathe for 2 minutes.

Relaxation Sequence 7

1. **Bound Angle Pose:** Sit up tall on your mat. Bring the soles of your feet together in front of you and let your knees drop out to the sides. Hold your feet in your hands and pull them in toward your inner thighs as far as you can comfortably. Bring your arms in flat against your torso and place your fingertips on the mat behind your hips. Take 10 full breaths (1 minute).

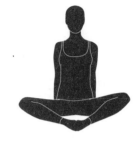

2. **Reclining Hand-to-Big-Toe Pose I:** Lie on your back and bring your knees into your chest. Grab your right big toe with your index and middle finger (or wrap a strap around the ball of your foot) and straighten out your leg in front of you as far as you can. Extend your left leg and keep your shoulders and head flat on the mat. Take 10 full breaths (1 minute). Repeat Reclining Hand-to-Big-Toe Pose I on the other side.

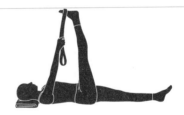

3. **Basic Relaxation Pose:** Extend your arms and legs flat on your mat. With your palms facing up, surrender to all effort and allow your body to melt into your mat. Let your muscles relax completely and allow all tension to drip off your fingertips and toes. Relax and breathe for 2 minutes.

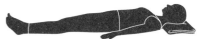

Relaxation Sequence 8

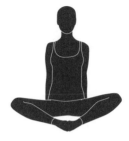

1. **Bound Angle Pose:** Sit up tall on your mat. Bring the soles of your feet together in front of you and let your knees drop out to the sides. Hold your feet in your hands and pull them in toward your inner thighs as far as you can comfortably. Bring your arms in flat against your torso and place your fingertips on the mat behind your hips. Take 10 full breaths (1 minute).

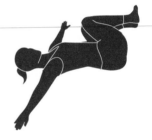

2. **Belly Twist:** Lie on your back and as you inhale, draw your knees into your chest. As you exhale, let your legs drop over to your left side, keeping your legs together and bent and your torso and arms flat on the mat. Twist your hips so your legs rest flat on the mat with your knees stacked on top of each other. Extend your arms out to the right and left in line with your shoulders and send your gaze over to the left for the full expression of this twist. Take 10 full breaths (1 minute). Repeat Belly Twist on the other side.

3. **Basic Relaxation Pose:** Extend your arms and legs flat on your mat. With your palms facing up, surrender to all effort and allow your body to melt into your mat. Let your muscles relax completely and allow all tension to drip off your fingertips and toes. Relax and breathe for 2 minutes.

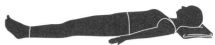

Relaxation Sequence 9

1. **Bound Angle Pose:** Sit up tall on your mat. Bring the soles of your feet together in front of you and let your knees drop out to the sides. Hold your feet in your hands and pull them in toward your inner thighs as far as you can comfortably. Bring your arms in flat against your torso and place your fingertips on the mat behind your hips. Take 10 full breaths (1 minute).

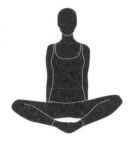

2. **Sage Twist:** Sit on your mat with your knees bent (place a folded blanket under your buttocks if it is more comfortable). Extend your left leg, place the fingertips of your right hand on the mat, and twist your torso to the right. Raise your left arm and press your elbow against the outside of your right upper thigh, near the knee, using this as leverage to twist your spine further and open your chest more. If you prefer, you can cross your right leg over the top of your left leg to enhance the twist. Take 10 full breaths (1 minute). Repeat Sage Twist on the other side.

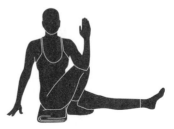

3. **Basic Relaxation Pose:** Lie flat on your mat and extend your arms and legs. With your palms facing up, surrender to all effort and allow your body to melt into your mat. Let your muscles relax completely and allow all tension to drip off your fingertips and toes. Relax and breathe for 2 minutes.

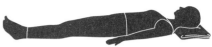

Relaxation Sequence 10

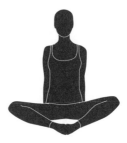

1. **Bound Angle Pose:** Sit up tall on your mat. Bring the soles of your feet together in front of you and let your knees drop out to the sides. Hold your feet in your hands and pull them in toward your inner thighs as far as you can comfortably. Bring your arms in flat against your torso and place your fingertips on the mat behind your hips. Take 10 full breaths (1 minute).

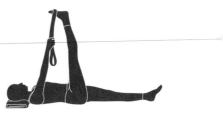

2. **Reclining Hand-to-Big-Toe Pose I:** Lie on your back and bring your knees into your chest. Grab your right big toe with your index and middle finger (or wrap a strap around the ball of your foot) and straighten out your leg in front of you as far as you can. Extend your left leg and keep your shoulders and head flat on the mat. Take 5 full breaths (30 seconds).

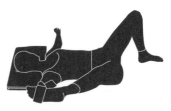

3. **Reclining Hand-to-Big-Toe Pose II:** Send your leg over to the side of your body and work to straighten the arm that is holding your toe. Take 5 full breaths (30 seconds). Repeat Reclining Hand-to-Big-Toe Pose I and II on the other side.

YOGA SEQUENCES FOR ACCEPTANCE

As you move through your day, you might encounter people, events, and situations that are confusing, disheartening, or frustrating. These poses help you accept what is around you without judgment. As you practice these sequences, you can mentally recite the mantra "It is what it is" and bring some serenity to your life.

Acceptance Sequence 1

1. **Downward-Facing Dog:** Exhale, plant your hands, and step your feet back behind you. Send your hips up high and fold your torso toward your thighs. Draw your thighs away from your kneecaps by engaging your quadriceps. Sink your heels toward the mat. Take 5 full breaths (30 seconds).

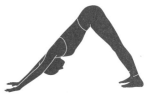

2. **Extended Side Angle Pose:** Inhale, then exhale and move one foot between your hands. Ground your back heel down, bend into your front knee, and twist from your lower torso as you reach your left hand up toward the ceiling. Keep your right hand on the floor next to your foot. Work to stack your shoulders on top of each other

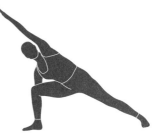

and spiral your ribs toward the ceiling. Reach up toward your top hand rather than down toward the ground. Take 5 full breaths (30 seconds).

3. **Revolved Side Angle Pose:** Keep your legs where they are, draw your left hand next to your right foot, and twist from your lower torso. Work to stack your shoulders on top of each other in the opposite direction. Take 5 full breaths (30 seconds). Repeat Extended Side Angle Pose and Revolved Side Angle Pose on the other side.

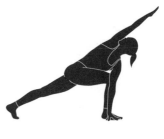

4. **Plank Pose:** Exhale, plant your hands palms down, shoulder-width apart, and extend your legs behind you. Place your feet hip-width apart with your toes pointed down. Create one long line of energy from your heels to the top of your head. Take 3 full breaths (15 seconds).

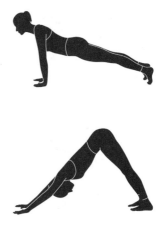

5. **Downward-Facing Dog:** Exhale, plant your hands, and step your feet back behind you. Send your hips up high and fold your torso toward your thighs. Draw your thighs away from your kneecaps by

engaging your quadriceps. Sink your heels toward the mat. Take 5 full breaths (30 seconds).

6. **Basic Relaxation Pose:** Lie flat on your mat and extend your arms and legs. With your palms facing up, surrender to all effort and allow your body to melt into your mat. Let your muscles relax completely and allow all tension to drip off your fingertips and toes. Relax and breathe for 1 minute.

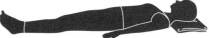

Acceptance Sequence 2

1. **Downward-Facing Dog:** Exhale, plant your hands, and step your feet back behind you. Send your hips up high and fold your torso toward your thighs. Draw your thighs away from your kneecaps by engaging your quadriceps. Sink your heels toward the mat. Take 5 full breaths (30 seconds).

2. **Triangle Pose:** Stand tall and walk your feet apart as far as you can comfortably. Turn your right foot in and rotate your left foot out, keeping your heels in line with each other. Exhale and extend laterally over your left leg, bending from the hip. Lower your left arm and place your fingertips lightly on your left shin or on the floor. Raise your right arm straight up, stacking your shoulders. Look straight ahead. Take 5 full breaths (30 seconds).

3. **Revolved Triangle Pose:** Keep your legs where they are, draw your left hand next to your right foot, and twist from your lower torso. Work to stack your shoulders on top of each other in the opposite

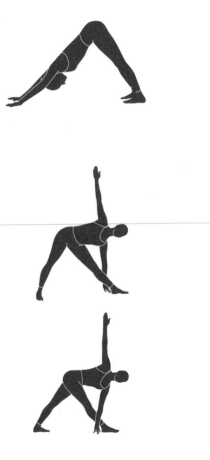

direction. Take 5 full breaths (30 seconds). Repeat Triangle Pose and Revolved Triangle Pose on the other side.

4. **Plank Pose:** Exhale, plant your hands palms down, shoulder-width apart, and extend your legs behind you. Place your feet hip-width apart with your toes pointed down. Create one long line of energy from your heels to the top of your head. Take 3 full breaths (15 seconds).

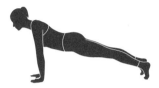

5. **Downward-Facing Dog:** Exhale, plant your hands, and step your feet back behind you. Send your hips up high and fold your torso toward your thighs. Draw your thighs away from your kneecaps by engaging your quadriceps. Sink your heels toward the mat. Take 5 full breaths (30 seconds).

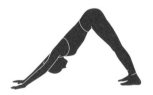

6. **Basic Relaxation Pose:** Lie flat on your mat and extend your arms and legs. With your palms facing up, surrender to all effort and allow your body to melt into your mat. Let your muscles relax completely and allow all tension to drip off your fingertips and toes. Relax and breathe for 1 minute.

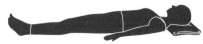

Acceptance Sequence 3

1. **Downward-Facing Dog:** Exhale, plant your hands, and step your feet back behind you. Send your hips up high and fold your torso toward your thighs. Draw your thighs away from your kneecaps by engaging your quadriceps. Sink your heels toward the mat. Take 5 full breaths (30 seconds).

2. **Equestrian Pose:** Inhale, then exhale and place your left foot between your hands. Inhale into the pose—drop down to your left knee and bring your fingertips to the floor directly under your shoulders. Work to stack your shoulders directly on top of your hips and open your chest. Take 5 breaths (30 seconds). Repeat Equestrian Pose on the other side.

3. **Intense Side Stretch Pose:** Exhale, keep your feet where they are, and hinge at your hips, leaning down toward your front leg. Keep your back and neck straight and lead with your chest. Fold your arms behind your back. Take 5 full breaths (30 seconds). Repeat Intense Side Stretch Pose on the other side.

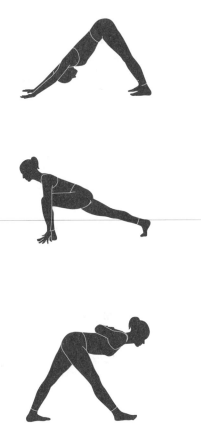

4. **Downward-Facing Dog:** Exhale, plant your hands, and step your feet back behind you. Send your hips up high and fold your torso toward your thighs. Draw your thighs away from your kneecaps by engaging your quadriceps. Sink your heels toward the mat. Take 5 full breaths (30 seconds).

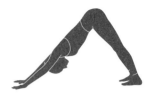

5. **Basic Relaxation Pose:** Lie flat on your mat and extend your arms and legs. With your palms facing up, surrender to all effort and allow your body to melt into your mat. Let your muscles relax completely and allow all tension to drip off your fingertips and toes. Relax and breathe for 1 minute.

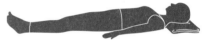

Acceptance Sequence 4

1. **Downward-Facing Dog:** Exhale, plant your hands, and step your feet back behind you. Send your hips up high and fold your torso toward your thighs. Draw your thighs away from your kneecaps by engaging your quadriceps. Sink your heels toward the mat. Take 5 full breaths (30 seconds).

2. **Cat-Cow:** Exhale and drop down to your hands and knees. Inhale, drop your belly, and arch your back, raising your tailbone. Lift your gaze as you find expansion across your chest. Exhale, arch your spine up, and lower your tailbone. Let your head hang heavy and look down between your thighs. Take 10 full breaths (1 minute).

3. **Child's Pose:** Exhale, kneel down on your mat, and bring your big toes together behind you. Spread out your knees and rest your torso on your thighs. Extend your arms above your head and rest your

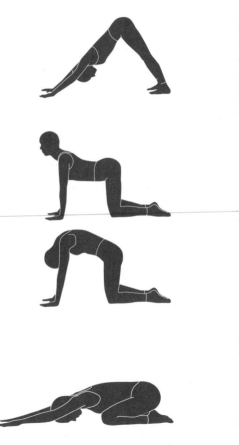

forehead on the mat. Spread your fingers evenly and wide. With every inhale, reach your fingertips toward the front of the mat and with every exhale, sink your hips closer to your heels. Take 10 full breaths (1 minute).

4. **Downward-Facing Dog:** Exhale, plant your hands, and step your feet back behind you. Send your hips up high and fold your torso toward your thighs. Draw your thighs away from your kneecaps by engaging your quadriceps. Sink your heels toward the mat. Take 5 full breaths (30 seconds).

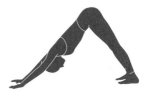

5. **Basic Relaxation Pose:** Lie flat on your mat and extend your arms and legs. With your palms facing up, surrender to all effort and allow your body to melt into your mat. Let your muscles relax completely and allow all tension to drip off your fingertips and toes. Relax and breathe for 1 minute.

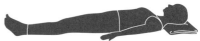

Acceptance Sequence 5

1. **Downward-Facing Dog:** Exhale, plant your hands, and step your feet back behind you. Send your hips up high and fold your torso toward your thighs. Draw your thighs away from your kneecaps by engaging your quadriceps. Sink your heels toward the mat. Take 5 full breaths (30 seconds).

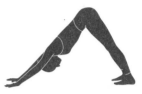

2. **Warrior I:** Inhale, then exhale and move one foot between your hands. Inhale into the position—ground your back heel down, bend your front knee into a 90-degree angle, stack your shoulders over your hips, and reach your arms straight up to the ceiling. Square your hips by drawing your front leg's outer hip back and pressing your opposite hip forward. Take 5 full breaths (30 seconds). Repeat Warrior I on the other side.

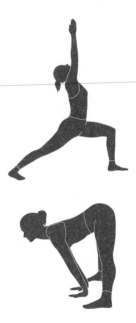

3. **Wide-Legged Forward Bend:** With your legs apart, pivot your toes in and your heels out. Extend your arms out to either side of your body and inhale. Exhale, hinge at your hips, and reach your hands palms down toward your mat with a flat back. Look forward as

you breathe, and then bend down further and let your head hang down. Come out of this pose the same way you came into it. Rise on an inhale with a flat back and your arms extended to your sides. Take 5 full breaths (30 seconds).

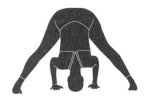

4. **Equestrian Pose:** Inhale, then exhale and place your left foot between your hands. Inhale into the pose—drop down to your left knee and bring your fingertips to the floor directly under your shoulders. Work to stack your shoulders directly on top of your hips and open your chest. Take 5 breaths (30 seconds). Repeat Equestrian Pose on the other side.

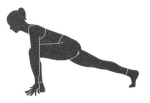

5. **Basic Relaxation Pose:** Lie flat on your mat and extend your arms and legs. With your palms facing up, surrender to all effort and allow your body to melt into your mat. Let your muscles relax completely and allow all tension to drip off your fingertips and toes. Relax and breathe for 1 minute.

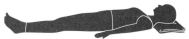

Acceptance Sequence 6

1. **Child's Pose:** Exhale, kneel down on your mat, and bring your big toes together behind you. Spread out your knees and rest your torso on your thighs. Extend your arms above your head and rest your forehead on the mat. Spread your fingers evenly and wide. With every inhale, reach your fingertips toward the front of the mat and with every exhale, sink your hips closer to your heels. Take 10 full breaths (1 minute).

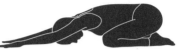

2. **Sphinx Pose:** Exhale, drop your hips down to the floor, and bring your elbows directly under your shoulders. Press your palms down into the floor and engage your legs. Find openness and release across your chest. Take 10 full breaths (1 minute).

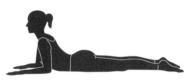

3. **Child's Pose:** Exhale, kneel down on your mat, and bring your big toes together behind you. Spread out your knees and rest your torso on your thighs. Extend your arms above your

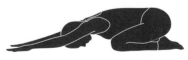

head and rest your forehead on the mat. Spread your fingers evenly and wide. With every inhale, reach your fingertips toward the front of the mat and with every exhale, sink your hips closer to your heels. Take 10 full breaths (1 minute).

4. **Basic Relaxation Pose:** Lie flat on your mat and extend your arms and legs. With your palms facing up, surrender to all effort and allow your body to melt into your mat. Let your muscles relax completely and allow all tension to drip off your fingertips and toes. Relax and breathe for 1 minute.

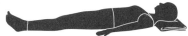

Acceptance Sequence 7

1. **Child's Pose:** Exhale, kneel down on your mat, and bring your big toes together behind you. Spread out your knees and rest your torso on your thighs. Extend your arms above your head and rest your forehead on the mat. Spread your fingers evenly and wide. With every inhale, reach your fingertips toward the front of the mat and with every exhale, sink your hips closer to your heels. Take 10 full breaths (1 minute).

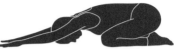

2. **Cat-Cow:** Exhale and drop down to your hands and knees. Inhale, drop your belly, and arch your back, raising your tailbone. Lift your gaze as you find expansion across your chest. Exhale, arch your spine up, and lower your tailbone. Let your head hang heavy and look down between your thighs. Take 10 full breaths (1 minute).

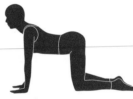

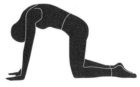

3. **Plank Pose:** Exhale, plant your hands palms down, shoulder-width apart, and extend your legs behind you. Place your feet hip-width apart with your toes pointed down. Create one long line of

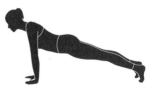

energy from your heels to the top of your head. Take 3 full breaths (15 seconds).

4. **Downward-Facing Dog:** Exhale, plant your hands, and step your feet back behind you. Send your hips up high and fold your torso toward your thighs. Draw your thighs away from your kneecaps by engaging your quadriceps. Sink your heels toward the mat. Take 5 full breaths (30 seconds).

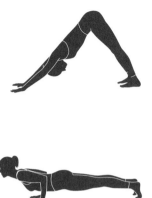

5. **Four-Limbed Staff Pose:** On your next exhale, bend your elbows and lower your entire body halfway to the mat. Keep your elbows close to your sides and make sure your elbows don't bend more than 90 degrees.

6. **Upward-Facing Dog:** For one breath in, press down through your palms, straighten your elbows, and open up through your chest. Stack your shoulders directly over your wrists and engage your legs enough to lift your knees and thighs away from your mat.

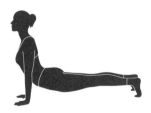

7. **Downward-Facing Dog:** Exhale, plant your hands, and step your feet back behind you. Send your hips up high and fold your torso toward your thighs. Draw your thighs away from your kneecaps by engaging your quadriceps. Sink your heels toward the mat. Take 5 full breaths (30 seconds).

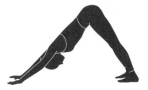

8. **Basic Relaxation Pose:** Lie flat on your mat and extend your arms and legs. With your palms facing up, surrender to all effort and allow your body to melt into your mat. Let your muscles relax completely and allow all tension to drip off your fingertips and toes. Relax and breathe for 1 minute.

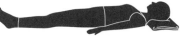

Acceptance Sequence 8

1. **Child's Pose:** Exhale, kneel down on your mat, and bring your big toes together behind you. Spread out your knees and rest your torso on your thighs. Extend your arms above your head and rest your forehead on the mat. Spread your fingers evenly and wide. With every inhale, reach your fingertips toward the front of the mat and with every exhale, sink your hips closer to your heels. Take 10 full breaths (1 minute).

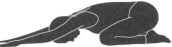

2. **Downward-Facing Dog:** Exhale, plant your hands, and step your feet back behind you. Send your hips up high and fold your torso toward your thighs. Draw your thighs away from your kneecaps by engaging your quadriceps. Sink your heels toward the mat. Take 5 full breaths (30 seconds).

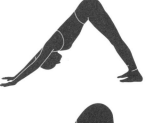

3. **Standing Forward Bend:** Exhale and hinge at your hips. Let your torso drape over your thighs and reach your fingers toward the ground, bending as far as you can comfortably to release your lower back. Take 10 full breaths (1 minute).

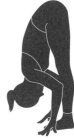

4. **Standing Half-Forward Bend:** For one breath in, place your hands on the chair in front of you and breathe. Create one line of energy from your tailbone to the top of your head. Plug your shoulders into their sockets and engage your shoulder blades together and down your back.

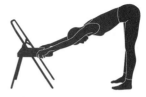

5. **Downward-Facing Dog:** Exhale, plant your hands, and step your feet back behind you. Send your hips up high and fold your torso toward your thighs. Draw your thighs away from your kneecaps by engaging your quadriceps. Sink your heels toward the mat. Take 5 full breaths (30 seconds).

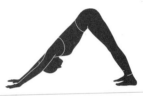

6. **Basic Relaxation Pose:** Lie flat on your mat and extend your arms and legs. With your palms facing up, surrender to all effort and allow your body to melt into your mat. Let your muscles relax completely and allow all tension to drip off your fingertips and toes. Relax and breathe for 1 minute.

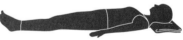

Acceptance Sequence 9

1. **Child's Pose:** Exhale, kneel down on your mat, and bring your big toes together behind you. Spread out your knees and rest your torso on your thighs. Extend [...] above your head and rest your [...]

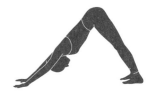

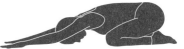

[...] palms down, shoulder-width [...] and extend your legs behind you. Place your feet hip-width apart with your toes pointed down. Create one long line of

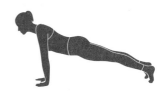

energy from your heels to the top of your head. Take 3 full breaths (15 seconds).

4. **Downward-Facing Dog:** Exhale, plant your hands, and step your feet back behind you. Send your hips up high and fold your torso toward your thighs. Draw your thighs away from your kneecaps by engaging your quadriceps. Sink your heels toward the mat. Take 5 full breaths (30 seconds).

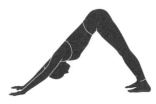

5. **Standing Forward Bend:** Exhale and hinge at your hips. Let your torso drape over your thighs and reach your fingers toward the ground, bending as far as you can comfortably to release your lower back. Take 5 full breaths (30 seconds).

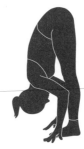

6. **Mountain Pose:** Stand tall, inhale, and reach your arms straight up to the ceiling. Ground down through the soles of your feet and squeeze your inner thighs together. Keep your lower ribs in and turn your pinkies inward to relax your shoulders away from your ears. Take 5 full breaths (30 seconds). Return your arms to your sides.

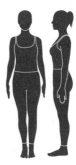

7. **Basic Relaxation Pose:** Lie flat on your mat and extend your arms and legs. With your palms facing up, surrender to all effort and allow your body to melt into your mat. Let your muscles relax completely and allow all tension to drip off your fingertips and toes. Relax and breathe for 1 minute.

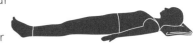

Acceptance Sequence 10

1. **Child's Pose:** Exhale, kneel down on your mat, and bring your big toes together behind you. Spread out your knees and rest your torso on your thighs. Extend your arms above your head and rest your forehead on the mat. Spread your fingers evenly and wide. With every inhale, reach your fingertips toward the front of the mat and with every exhale, sink your hips closer to your heels. Take 10 full breaths (1 minute).

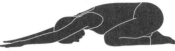

2. **Downward-Facing Dog:** Exhale, plant your hands, and step your feet back behind you. Send your hips up high and fold your torso toward your thighs. Draw your thighs away from your kneecaps by engaging your quadriceps. Sink your heels toward the mat. Take 5 full breaths (30 seconds).

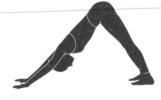

3. **Salute with Eight Parts:** Exhale, drop your knees to the mat, and then lower your chest to the mat. Keep your hands directly underneath your shoulders and rest your chin on the mat as you gaze forward. Take 5 full breaths (30 seconds).

4. **Child's Pose:** Exhale, kneel down on your mat, and bring your big toes together behind you. Spread out your knees and rest your torso on your thighs. Extend your arms above your head and rest your forehead on the mat. Spread your fingers evenly and wide. With every inhale, reach your fingertips toward the front of the mat and with every exhale, sink your hips closer to your heels. Take 10 full breaths (1 minute).

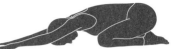

5. **Plank Pose:** Exhale, plant your hands palms down, shoulder-width apart, and extend your legs behind you. Place your feet hip-width apart with your toes pointed down. Create one long line of energy from your heels to the top of your head. Take 3 full breaths (15 seconds).

6. **Cobra Pose:** Exhale, lower down to your belly, bring your hands directly underneath your shoulders by your lower ribs, and bring your legs together. On an inhale, peel your chest away from the mat using your body and putting little to no weight on your hands. Straighten out

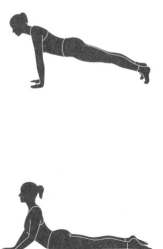

your legs and stretch your chest forward with your hands palms down, arms lightly bent at the elbow, and your chest and head aligned. Take 5 full breaths (30 seconds).

7. **Child's Pose:** Exhale, kneel down on your mat, and bring your big toes together behind you. Spread out your knees and rest your torso on your thighs. Extend your arms above your head and rest your forehead on the mat. Spread your fingers evenly and wide. With every inhale, reach your fingertips toward the front of the mat and with every exhale, sink your hips closer to your heels. Take 5 full breaths (30 seconds).

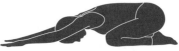

8. **Basic Relaxation Pose:** Lie flat on your mat and extend your arms and legs. With your palms facing up, surrender to all effort and allow your body to melt into your mat. Let your muscles relax completely and allow all tension to drip off your fingertips and toes. Relax and breathe for 30 seconds.

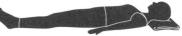

YOGA SEQUENCES FOR RELEASE

Once you have accepted what is around you without judgment, you can release your fears and worries into the universe. These sequences will lift the weight off your shoulders and give you the motivation to improve your well-being and that of those around you.

Release Sequence 1

1. **Downward-Facing Dog:** Exhale, plant your hands, and step your feet back behind you. Send your hips up high and fold your torso toward your thighs. Draw your thighs away from your kneecaps by engaging your quadriceps. Sink your heels toward the mat. Take 20 full breaths (2 minutes).

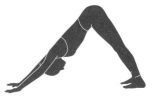

2. **Bridge Pose:** Lie down on your back, bend your knees, and place your feet a bit more than hip-width apart, flat on the mat. Inhale as you raise your hips. Exhale, shimmy your shoulders underneath you, and extend your arms, clenching your hands into fists. Breathe air into your belly and find space across your chest. Take 10 full breaths (1 minute).

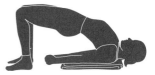

3. **Basic Relaxation Pose:** Lie flat on your mat and extend your arms and legs. With your palms facing up, surrender to all effort and allow your body to melt into your mat. Let your muscles relax completely and allow all tension to drip off your fingertips and toes. Relax and breathe for 2 minutes.

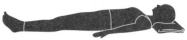

Release Sequence 2

1. **Downward-Facing Dog:** Exhale, plant your hands, and step your feet back behind you. Send your hips up high and fold your torso toward your thighs. Draw your thighs away from your kneecaps by engaging your quadriceps. Sink your heels toward the mat. Take 20 full breaths (2 minutes).

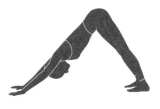

2. **Bridge Pose:** Lie down on your back, bend your knees, and place your feet a bit more than hip-width apart, flat on the mat. Inhale as you raise your hips. Exhale, shimmy your shoulders underneath you, and extend your arms, clenching your hands into fists. Breathe air into your belly and find space across your chest. Take 10 full breaths (1 minute).

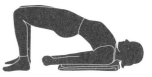

3. **Basic Relaxation Pose:** Lie flat on your mat and extend your arms and legs. With your palms facing up, surrender to all effort and allow your body to melt into your mat. Let your muscles relax completely and allow all tension to drip off your fingertips and toes. Relax and breathe for 2 minutes.

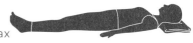

Release Sequence 3

1. **Downward-Facing Dog:** Exhale, plant your hands, and step your feet back behind you. Send your hips up high and fold your torso toward your thighs. Draw your thighs away from your kneecaps by engaging your quadriceps. Sink your heels toward the mat. Take 3 full breaths (15 seconds).

2. **Warrior II:** Inhale as you move into Warrior II—ground your back heel down and move your hips to open along with your chest. Lower your arms to extend outward from your shoulders to your fingertips. Bend into your front knee up to 90 degrees and make sure it's stacked directly over your ankle. Keep your back leg engaged and externally rotate your front thigh. Take 5 full breaths (30 seconds). Repeat Warrior II on the other side.

3. **Triangle Pose:** Exhale, keep your feet where they are, straighten your front knee, and twist from your lower torso as you reach your top hand up toward the ceiling and your other hand to the mat. Work to stack

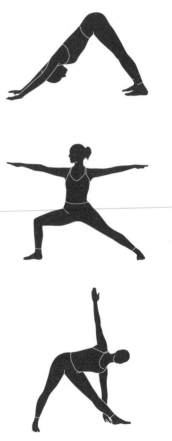

your shoulders on top of each other and spiral your ribs toward the ceiling. Reach up toward your top hand rather than down toward the ground. Take 5 full breaths (30 seconds).

4. **Wide-Legged Forward Bend:** With your legs apart, pivot your toes in and your heels out. Extend your arms out to either side of your body and inhale. Exhale, hinge at your hips, and reach your hands palms down toward your mat with a flat back. Look forward as you breathe, and then bend down further and let your head hang down. Come out of this pose the same way you came into it. Rise on an inhale with a flat back and your arms extended to your sides. Take 5 full breaths (30 seconds).

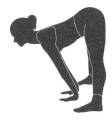

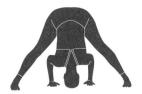

Release Sequence 4

1. **Downward-Facing Dog:** Exhale, plant your hands, and step your feet back behind you. Send your hips up high and fold your torso toward your thighs. Draw your thighs away from your kneecaps by engaging your quadriceps. Sink your heels toward the mat. Take 10 full breaths (1 minute).

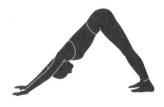

2. **Reclining Hero Pose:** Exhale and drop down to your knees, leaning back onto your heels (place folded blankets or bolsters underneath your torso and head if necessary to prop yourself). If it feels comfortable, allow your feet to come to the outside of your thighs. Drop your arms to your sides. Either stay in this position or make your way all the way down to your back. If this feels comfortable, bring your arms above your head and grab opposite elbows for the full expression of the pose. Take 20 full breaths (2 minutes).

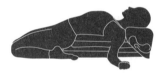

3. **Basic Relaxation Pose:** Lie flat on your
   mat and extend your arms and legs.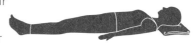
   With your palms facing up, surrender
   to all effort and allow your body to
   melt into your mat. Let your muscles relax
   completely and allow all tension to drip
   off your fingertips and toes. Relax and
   breathe for 2 minutes.

Release Sequence 5

1. **Downward-Facing Dog:** Exhale, plant your hands, and step your feet back behind you. Send your hips up high and fold your torso toward your thighs. Draw your thighs away from your kneecaps by engaging your quadriceps. Sink your heels toward the mat. Take 10 full breaths (1 minute).

2. **Cat-Cow:** Exhale and drop down to your hands and knees. Inhale, drop your belly, and arch your back, raising your tailbone. Lift your gaze as you find expansion across your chest. Exhale, arch your spine up, and lower your tailbone. Let your head hang heavy and look down between your thighs. Take 10 full breaths (1 minute).

3. **Reclining Hero Pose:** Exhale and drop down to your knees, leaning back onto your heels (place folded blankets or bolsters underneath your torso and head if necessary to prop yourself). If it feels comfortable, allow your feet to come to the outside of your thighs. Drop your

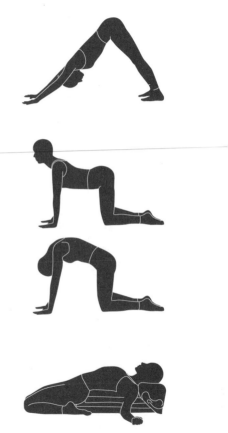

arms to your sides. Either stay in this position or make your way all the way down to your back. If this feels comfortable, bring your arms above your head and grab opposite elbows for the full expression of the pose. Take 20 full breaths (2 minutes).

4. **Basic Relaxation Pose:** Lie flat on your mat and extend your arms and legs. 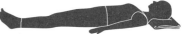 With your palms facing up, surrender to all effort and allow your body to melt into your mat. Let your muscles relax completely and allow all tension to drip off your fingertips and toes. Relax and breathe for 1 minute.

Release Sequence 6

1. **Downward-Facing Dog:** Exhale, plant your hands, and step your feet back behind you. Send your hips up high and fold your torso toward your thighs. Draw your thighs away from your kneecaps by engaging your quadriceps. Sink your heels toward the mat. Take 10 full breaths (1 minute).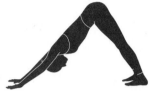

2. **Bound Angle Pose:** Sit up tall on your mat. Bring the soles of your feet together in front of you and let your knees drop out to the sides. Hold your feet in your hands and pull them in toward your inner thighs as far as you can comfortably. Bring your arms in flat against your torso and place your fingertips on the mat behind your hips. Take 20 full breaths (2 minutes).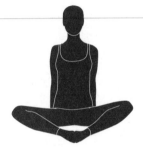

3. **Basic Relaxation Pose:** Lie flat on your mat and extend your arms and legs. With your palms facing up, surrender to all effort and allow your body to melt into your mat. Let your muscles relax completely and allow all tension to drip off your fingertips and toes. Relax and breathe for 2 minutes.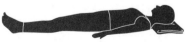

Release Sequence 7

1. **Downward-Facing Dog:** Exhale, plant your hands, and step your feet back behind you. Send your hips up high and fold your torso toward your thighs. Draw your thighs away from your kneecaps by engaging your quadriceps. Sink your heels toward the mat. Take 10 full breaths (1 minute).

2. **Standing Forward Bend:** Exhale and hinge at your hips. Let your torso drape over your thighs and reach your fingers toward the ground, bending as far as you can comfortably to release your lower back. Take 10 full breaths (1 minute).

3. **Downward-Facing Dog:** Exhale, plant your hands, and step your feet back behind you. Send your hips up high and fold your torso toward your thighs. Draw your thighs away from your kneecaps by engaging your quadriceps. Sink your heels toward the mat. Take 10 full breaths (1 minute).

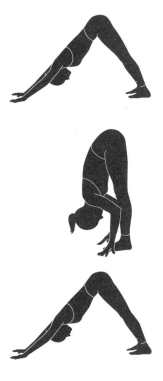

4. **Basic Relaxation Pose:** Lie flat on your mat and extend your arms and legs. With your palms facing up, surrender to all effort and allow your body to melt into your mat. Let your muscles relax completely and allow all tension to drip off your fingertips and toes. Relax and breathe for 2 minutes.

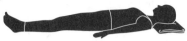

Release Sequence 8

1. **Downward-Facing Dog:** Exhale, plant your hands, and step your feet back behind you. Send your hips up high and fold your torso toward your thighs. Draw your thighs away from your kneecaps by engaging your quadriceps. Sink your heels toward the mat. Take 10 full breaths (1 minute).

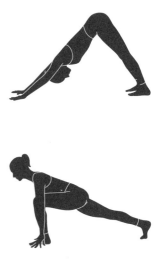

2. **Equestrian Pose:** Inhale, then exhale and place your left foot between your hands. Inhale into the pose—drop down to your left knee and bring your fingertips to the floor directly under your shoulders. Work to stack your shoulders directly on top of your hips and open your chest. Take 10 full breaths (1 minute). Repeat Equestrian Pose on the other side.

3. **Basic Relaxation Pose:** Lie flat on your mat and extend your arms and legs. With your palms facing up, surrender to all effort and allow your body to melt into your mat. Let your muscles relax completely and allow all tension to drip off your fingertips and toes. Relax and breathe for 2 minutes.

Release Sequence 9

1. **Downward-Facing Dog:** Exhale, plant your hands, and step your feet back behind you. Send your hips up high and fold your torso toward your thighs. Draw your thighs away from your kneecaps by engaging your quadriceps. Sink your heels toward the mat. Take 10 full breaths (1 minute).

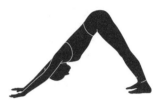

2. **Plank Pose:** Exhale, plant your hands palms down, shoulder-width apart, and extend your legs behind you. Place your feet hip-width apart with your toes pointed down. Create one long line of energy from your heels to the top of your head. Take 3 full breaths (15 seconds). Inhale.

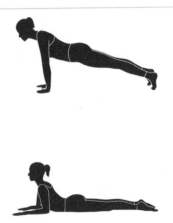

3. **Sphinx Pose:** Exhale, drop your hips down to the floor, and bring your elbows directly under your shoulders. Press your palms down into the floor and engage your legs. Find openness and release across your chest. Take 10 full breaths (1 minute).

4. **Child's Pose:** Exhale, kneel down on your mat, and bring your big toes together behind you. Spread out your knees and rest your torso on your thighs. Extend your arms above your head and rest your forehead on the mat. Spread your fingers evenly and wide. With every inhale, reach your fingertips toward the front of the mat and with every exhale, sink your hips closer to your heels. Take 10 full breaths (1 minute).

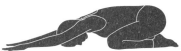

5. **Downward-Facing Dog:** Exhale, plant your hands, and step your feet back behind you. Send your hips up high and fold your torso toward your thighs. Draw your thighs away from your kneecaps by engaging your quadriceps. Sink your heels toward the mat. Take 3 full breaths (15 seconds).

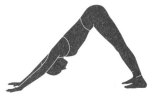

6. **Basic Relaxation Pose:** Lie flat on your mat and extend your arms and legs. With your palms facing up, surrender to all effort and allow your body to melt into your mat. Let your muscles relax completely and allow all tension to drip off your fingertips and toes. Relax and breathe for 1 minute.

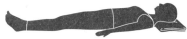

Release Sequence 10

1. **Downward-Facing Dog:** Exhale, plant your hands, and step your feet back behind you. Send your hips up high and fold your torso toward your thighs. Draw your thighs away from your kneecaps by engaging your quadriceps. Sink your heels toward the mat. Take 5 full breaths (30 seconds).

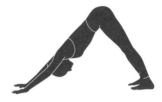

2. **Standing Forward Bend:** Exhale and hinge at your hips. Let your torso drape over your thighs and reach your fingers toward the ground, bending as far as you can comfortably to release your lower back. Take 5 full breaths (30 seconds).

3. **Chair Pose:** Inhale, bend your knees, and sweep your arms up toward the ceiling. Sink your weight into your hips and let the weight sink all the way down into your heels. Squeeze your inner thighs together, keep your lower ribs in, and relax your shoulders away from your ears. Take 5 full breaths (30 seconds).

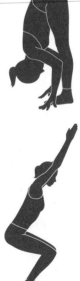

4. **Chair Twist:** Sit down sideways on a chair. Exhale and bring your palms to prayer at your heart center. Twist your torso toward the back of the chair, bringing your right elbow to the outside of your right thigh and grasping the back of the chair. Grasp the other side of the chair back with your other hand. Use your arms as leverage to peel your torso away from your thighs and twist open even more. Take 5 full breaths (30 seconds). Repeat Chair Twist on the other side.

5. **Chair Pose:** Inhale, bend your knees, and sweep your arms up toward the ceiling. Sink your weight into your hips and let the weight sink all the way down into your heels. Squeeze your inner thighs together, keep your lower ribs in, and relax your shoulders away from your ears. Take 5 full breaths (30 seconds).

6. **Standing Forward Bend:** Exhale and hinge at your hips. Let your torso drape over your thighs and reach your fingers toward the ground, bending as far as you can comfortably to release your lower back. Take 3 full breaths (15 seconds).

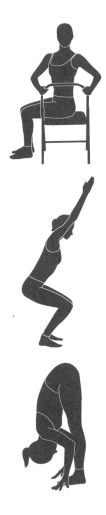

7. **Basic Relaxation Pose:** Lie flat on your mat and extend your arms and legs. With your palms facing up, surrender to all effort and allow your body to melt into your mat. Let your muscles relax completely and allow all tension to drip off your fingertips and toes. Relax and breathe for 1 minute.

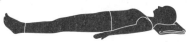

SEQUENCES
BODY

YOGA SEQUENCES FOR ENERGY

Though yoga can be a serene, quiet experience, it can also enliven your muscles and boost your energy level as well. The following sequences are perfect for an early-morning practice to get your day going, or for a late-afternoon pick-me-up instead of having another cup of coffee.

Energy Sequence 1

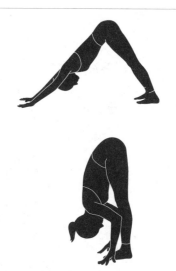

1. **Downward-Facing Dog:** Exhale, plant your hands, and step your feet back behind you. Send your hips up high and fold your torso toward your thighs. Draw your thighs away from your kneecaps by engaging your quadriceps. Sink your heels toward the mat. Take 10 full breaths (1 minute).

2. **Standing Forward Bend:** Exhale and hinge at your hips. Let your torso drape over your thighs and reach your fingers toward the ground, bending as far as you can comfortably to release your lower back. Take 3 full breaths (15 seconds).

3. **Mountain Pose:** Stand tall, inhale, and reach your arms straight up to the ceiling. Ground down through the soles of your feet and squeeze your inner thighs together. Keep your lower ribs in and turn your pinkies inward to relax your shoulders away from your ears. Take 5 full breaths (30 seconds). Return your arms to your sides.

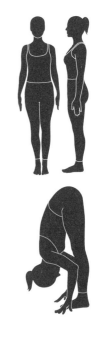

4. **Standing Forward Bend:** Exhale and hinge at your hips. Let your torso drape over your thighs and reach your fingers toward the ground, bending as far as you can comfortably to release your lower back. Take 3 full breaths (15 seconds).

5. **Plank Pose:** Exhale, plant your hands palms down, shoulder-width apart, and extend your legs behind you. Place your feet hip-width apart with your toes pointed down. Create one long line of energy from your heels to the top of your head. Take 5 full breaths (30 seconds).

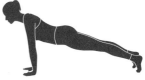

6. **Four-Limbed Staff Pose:** On your next exhale, bend your elbows and lower your entire body halfway to the mat. Keep your elbows close to your sides and make sure your elbows don't bend more than 90 degrees.

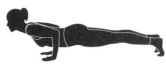

7. **Upward-Facing Dog:** For one breath in, press down through your palms, straighten your elbows, and open up through your chest. Stack your shoulders directly over your wrists and engage your legs enough to lift your knees and thighs away from your mat.

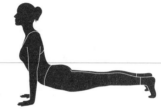

8. **Downward-Facing Dog:** Exhale, plant your hands, and step your feet back behind you. Send your hips up high and fold your torso toward your thighs. Draw your thighs away from your kneecaps by engaging your quadriceps. Sink your heels toward the mat. Take 20 full breaths (2 minutes).

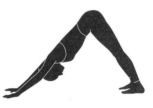

Energy Sequence 2

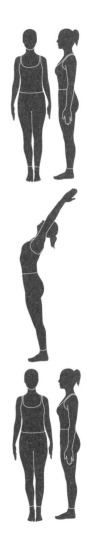

1. **Mountain Pose:** Stand tall, inhale, and reach your arms straight up. Ground through the soles of your feet and squeeze your inner thighs together. Keep your lower ribs in and turn your pinkies inward to relax your shoulders away from your ears. Take 10 full breaths (1 minute). Return your arms to your sides.

2. **Standing Backbend Pose:** Exhale, bring your palms together over your head, and look up toward your thumbs. Stretch up from your hips as you arch slightly at the top of your back. Make this intentionally exploratory without forcing anything. Take 3 full breaths (15 seconds).

3. **Mountain Pose:** Stand tall, inhale, and reach your arms straight up. Ground through the soles of your feet and squeeze your inner thighs together. Keep your lower ribs in and turn your pinkies inward to relax your shoulders away from your ears. Take 3 full breaths (15 seconds). Return your arms to your sides.

4. **Standing Forward Bend:** Exhale and hinge at your hips. Let your torso drape over your thighs and reach your fingers toward the ground, bending as far as you can comfortably to release your lower back. Take 5 full breaths (30 seconds).

5. **Standing Half-Forward Bend:** For one breath in, place your hands on the chair in front of you and breathe. Create one line of energy from your tailbone to the top of your head. Plug your shoulders into their sockets and engage your shoulder blades together and down your back.

6. **Plank Pose:** Exhale, plant your hands palms down, shoulder-width apart, and extend your legs behind you. Place your feet hip-width apart with your toes pointed down. Create one long line of energy from your heels to the top of your head. Take 5 full breaths (30 seconds).

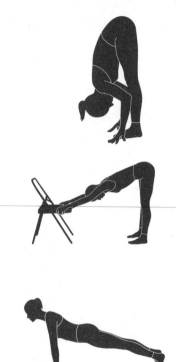

7. **Downward-Facing Dog:** Exhale, plant your hands, and step your feet back behind you. Send your hips up high and fold your torso toward your thighs. Draw your thighs away from your kneecaps by engaging your quadriceps. Sink your heels toward the mat. Take 20 full breaths (2 minutes).

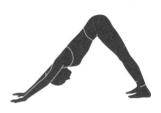

Energy Sequence 3

1. **Downward-Facing Dog:** Exhale, plant your hands, and step your feet back behind you. Send your hips up high and fold your torso toward your thighs. Draw your thighs away from your kneecaps by engaging your quadriceps. Sink your heels toward the mat. Take 20 full breaths (2 minutes).

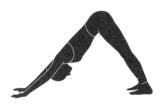

2. **Plank Pose:** Exhale, plant your hands palms down, shoulder-width apart, and extend your legs behind you. Place your feet hip-width apart with your toes pointed down. Create one long line of energy from your heels to the top of your head. Take 5 full breaths (30 seconds).

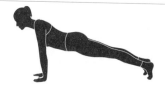

3. **Salute with Eight Parts or Points:** Exhale, drop your knees to the mat, and then lower your chest to the mat. Keep your hands directly underneath your shoulders and rest your chin on the mat as you gaze forward. Take 5 full breaths (30 seconds).

4. **Cobra Pose:** Exhale, lower down to your belly, bring your hands directly underneath your shoulders by your lower ribs, and bring your legs together. On an inhale, peel your chest away from the mat using your body and putting little to no weight on your hands. Straighten out your legs and stretch your chest forward with your hands palms down, arms lightly bent at the elbow, and your chest and head aligned. Take 5 full breaths (30 seconds).

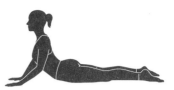

5. **Plank Pose:** Inhale and press into your palms to slowly lift your body by straightening your arms. Create one long line of energy from your heels to the top of your head. Take 5 full breaths (30 seconds).

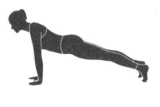

6. **Downward-Facing Dog:** Exhale, plant your hands, and step your feet back behind you. Send your hips up high and fold your torso toward your thighs. Draw your thighs away from your kneecaps by engaging your quadriceps. Sink your heels toward the mat. Take 10 full breaths (1 minute).

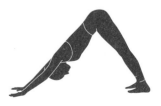

Energy Sequence 4

1. **Downward-Facing Dog:** Exhale, plant your hands, and step your feet back behind you. Send your hips up high and fold your torso toward your thighs. Draw your thighs away from your kneecaps by engaging your quadriceps. Sink your heels toward the mat. Take 10 full breaths (1 minute).

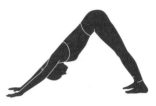

2. **Standing Forward Bend:** Exhale and hinge at your hips. Let your torso drape over your thighs and reach your fingers toward the ground, bending as far as you can comfortably to release your lower back. Take 5 full breaths (30 seconds).

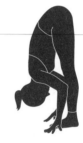

3. **Standing Half-Forward Bend:** For one breath in, place your hands on the chair in front of you and breathe. Create one line of energy from your tailbone to the top of your head. Plug your shoulders into their sockets and engage your shoulder blades together and down your back. Take 5 full breaths (30 seconds).

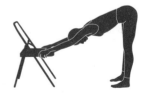

4. **Standing Forward Bend:** Exhale and hinge at your hips. Let your torso drape over your thighs and reach your fingers toward the ground, bending as far as you can comfortably to release your lower back.

5. **Mountain Pose:** Stand tall, inhale, and reach your arms straight up to the ceiling. Ground down through the soles of your feet and squeeze your inner thighs together. Keep your lower ribs in and turn your pinkies inward to relax your shoulders away from your ears. Take 5 full breaths (30 seconds). Return your arms to your sides.

6. **Standing Forward Bend:** Exhale and hinge at your hips. Let your torso drape over your thighs and reach your fingers toward the ground, bending as far as you can comfortably to release your lower back.

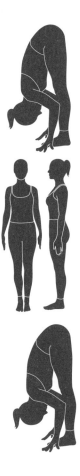

7. **Standing Half-Forward Bend:** For one breath in, place your hands on the chair in front of you and breathe. Create one line of energy from your tailbone to the top of your head. Plug your shoulders into their sockets and engage your shoulder blades together and down your back.

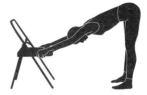

8. **Plank Pose:** Exhale, plant your hands palms down, shoulder-width apart, and extend your legs behind you. Place your feet hip-width apart with your toes pointed down. Create one long line of energy from your heels to the top of your head. Take 5 full breaths (30 seconds).

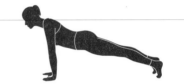

9. **Downward-Facing Dog:** Exhale, plant your hands, and step your feet back behind you. Send your hips up high and fold your torso toward your thighs. Draw your thighs away from your kneecaps by engaging your quadriceps. Sink your heels toward the mat. Take 10 full breaths (1 minute).

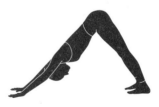

Energy Sequence 5

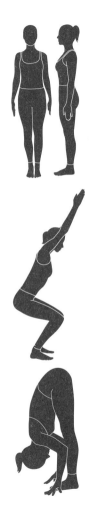

1. **Mountain Pose:** Stand tall, inhale, and reach your arms straight up to the ceiling. Ground down through the soles of your feet and squeeze your inner thighs together. Keep your lower ribs in and turn your pinkies inward to relax your shoulders away from your ears. Take 10 full breaths (1 minute). Return your arms to your sides.

2. **Chair Pose:** Inhale, bend your knees, and sweep your arms up toward the ceiling. Sink your weight into your hips and let the weight sink all the way down into your heels. Squeeze your inner thighs together, keep your lower ribs in, and relax your shoulders away from your ears. Take 5 full breaths (30 seconds).

3. **Standing Forward Bend:** Exhale and hinge at your hips. Let your torso drape over your thighs and reach your fingers toward the ground, bending as far as you can comfortably to release your lower back. Take 5 full breaths (30 seconds).

4. **Standing Half-Forward Bend:** For one breath in, place your hands on the chair in front of you and breathe. Create one line of energy from your tailbone to the top of your head. Plug your shoulders into their sockets and engage your shoulder blades together and down your back.

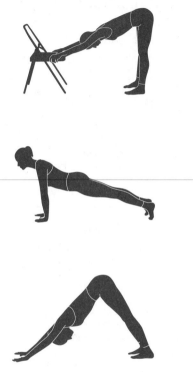

5. **Plank Pose:** Exhale, plant your hands palms down, shoulder-width apart, and extend your legs behind you. Place your feet hip-width apart with your toes pointed down. Create one long line of energy from your heels to the top of your head. Take 10 full breaths (1 minute).

6. **Downward-Facing Dog:** Exhale, plant your hands, and step your feet back behind you. Send your hips up high and fold your torso toward your thighs. Draw your thighs away from your kneecaps by engaging your quadriceps. Sink your heels toward the mat. Take 10 full breaths (1 minute).

Energy Sequence 6

1. **Downward-Facing Dog:** Exhale, plant your hands, and step your feet back behind you. Send your hips up high and fold your torso toward your thighs. Draw your thighs away from your kneecaps by engaging your quadriceps. Sink your heels toward the mat. Take 10 full breaths (1 minute).

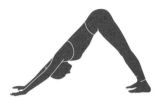

2. **Standing Forward Bend:** Exhale and hinge at your hips. Let your torso drape over your thighs and reach your fingers toward the ground, bending as far as you can comfortably to release your lower back. Take 5 full breaths (30 seconds).

3. **Chair Pose:** Inhale, bend your knees, and sweep your arms up toward the ceiling. Sink your weight into your hips and let the weight sink all the way down into your heels. Squeeze your inner thighs together, keep your lower ribs in, and relax your shoulders away from your ears. Take 5 full breaths (30 seconds).

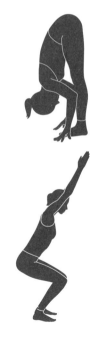

153

4. **Plank Pose:** Exhale, plant your hands palms down, shoulder-width apart, and extend your legs behind you. Place your feet hip-width apart with your toes pointed down. Create one long line of energy from your heels to the top of your head. Take 3 full breaths (15 seconds).

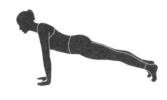

5. **Four-Limbed Staff Pose:** On your next exhale, bend your elbows and lower your entire body halfway to the mat. Keep your elbows close to your sides and make sure your elbows don't bend more than 90 degrees.

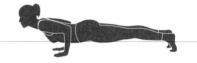

6. **Upward-Facing Dog:** On your next breath in, press down through your palms, straighten your elbows, and open up through your chest. Stack your shoulders directly over your wrists and engage your legs enough to lift your knees and thighs away from your mat.

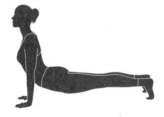

7. **Downward-Facing Dog:** Exhale, plant your hands, and step your feet back behind you. Send your hips up high and fold your torso toward your thighs. Draw your thighs away from your kneecaps by engaging your quadriceps. Sink your heels toward the mat. Take 10 full breaths (1 minute).

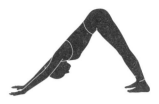

Energy Sequence 7

1. **Downward-Facing Dog:** Exhale, plant your hands, and step your feet back behind you. Send your hips up high and fold your torso toward your thighs. Draw your thighs away from your kneecaps by engaging your quadriceps. Sink your heels toward the mat. Take 5 full breaths (30 seconds).

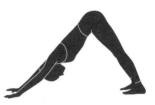

2. **Warrior I:** Inhale, then exhale and move one foot between your hands. Inhale into the position—ground your back heel down, bend your front knee into a 90-degree angle, stack your shoulders over your hips, and reach your arms straight up to the ceiling. Square your hips by drawing your front leg's outer hip back and pressing your opposite hip forward. Take 5 full breaths (30 seconds). Repeat Warrior I on the other side.

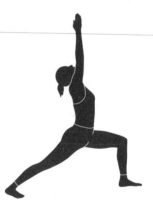

3. **Plank Pose:** Exhale, plant your hands palms down, shoulder-width apart, and extend your legs behind you. Place your feet hip-width apart with your toes pointed down. Create one long line of energy from your

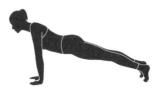

heels to the top of your head. Take 5 full
breaths (30 seconds).

4. **Four-Limbed Staff Pose:** On your next
   exhale, bend your elbows and lower
   your entire body halfway to the mat.
   Keep your elbows close to your sides
   and make sure your elbows don't bend
   more than 90 degrees.

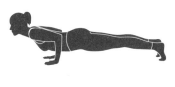

5. **Upward-Facing Dog:** On your next
   breath in, press down through your
   palms, straighten your elbows, and
   open up through your chest. Stack your
   shoulders directly over your wrists and
   engage your legs enough to lift your
   knees and thighs away from your mat.

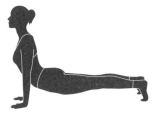

6. **Downward-Facing Dog:** Exhale, plant
   your hands, and step your feet back
   behind you. Send your hips up high and
   fold your torso toward your thighs. Draw
   your thighs away from your kneecaps
   by engaging your quadriceps. Sink your
   heels toward the mat. Take 5 full breaths
   (30 seconds).

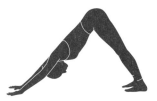

Energy Sequence 8

1. **Downward-Facing Dog:** Exhale, plant your hands, and step your feet back behind you. Send your hips up high and fold your torso toward your thighs. Draw your thighs away from your kneecaps by engaging your quadriceps. Sink your heels toward the mat. Take 5 full breaths (30 seconds).

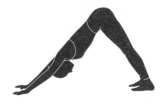

2. **Warrior II:** Inhale as you move into Warrior II—ground your back heel down and move your hips to open along with your chest. Lower your arms to extend outward from your shoulders to your fingertips. Bend into your front knee up to 90 degrees and make sure it's stacked directly over your ankle. Keep your back leg engaged and externally rotate your front thigh. Take 5 full breaths (30 seconds). Repeat Warrior II on the other side.

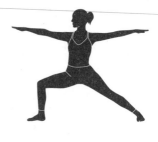

3. **Plank Pose:** Exhale, plant your hands palms down, shoulder-width apart, and extend your legs behind you. Place your feet hip-width apart with your toes pointed down. Create one long line of energy from your

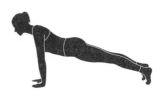

heels to the top of your head. Take 3 full breaths (15 seconds).

4. **Four-Limbed Staff Pose:** On your next exhale, bend your elbows and lower your entire body halfway to the mat. Keep your elbows close to your sides and make sure your elbows don't bend more than 90 degrees.

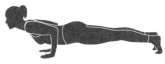

5. **Upward-Facing Dog:** On your next breath in, press down through your palms, straighten your elbows, and open up through your chest. Stack your shoulders directly over your wrists and engage your legs enough to lift your knees and thighs away from your mat.

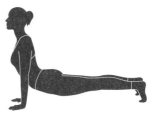

6. **Downward-Facing Dog:** Exhale, plant your hands, and step your feet back behind you. Send your hips up high and fold your torso toward your thighs. Draw your thighs away from your kneecaps by engaging your quadriceps. Sink your heels toward the mat. Take 5 full breaths (30 seconds).

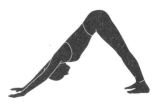

Energy Sequence 9

1. **Downward-Facing Dog:** Exhale, plant your hands, and step your feet back behind you. Send your hips up high and fold your torso toward your thighs. Draw your thighs away from your kneecaps by engaging your quadriceps. Sink your heels toward the mat. Take 5 full breaths (30 seconds).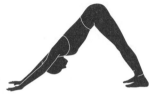

2. **Triangle Pose:** Stand tall and walk your feet apart as far as you can comfortably. Turn your right foot in and rotate your left foot out, keeping your heels in line with each other. Exhale and extend laterally over your left leg, bending from the hip. Lower your left arm and place your fingertips lightly on your left shin or on the floor. Raise your right arm straight up, stacking your shoulders. Look straight ahead. Take 5 full breaths (30 seconds). Repeat Triangle Pose on the other side.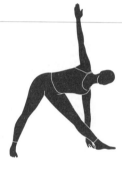

3. **Plank Pose:** Exhale, plant your hands palms down, shoulder-width apart, and extend your legs behind you. Place your feet hip-width apart with your toes pointed down.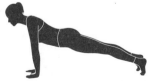

Create one long line of energy from your heels to the top of your head. Take 3 full breaths (15 seconds).

4. **Four-Limbed Staff Pose:** On your next exhale, bend your elbows and lower your entire body halfway to the mat. Keep your elbows close to your sides and make sure your elbows don't bend more than 90 degrees.

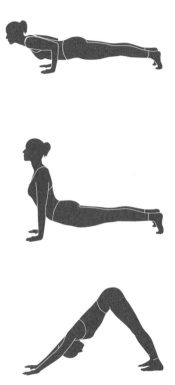

5. **Upward-Facing Dog:** On your next breath in, press down through your palms, straighten your elbows, and open up through your chest. Stack your shoulders directly over your wrists and engage your legs enough to lift your knees and thighs away from your mat.

6. **Downward-Facing Dog:** Exhale, plant your hands, and step your feet back behind you. Send your hips up high and fold your torso toward your thighs. Draw your thighs away from your kneecaps by engaging your quadriceps. Sink your heels toward the mat. Take 3 full breaths (15 seconds).

Energy Sequence 10

1. **Downward-Facing Dog:** Exhale, plant your hands, and step your feet back behind you. Send your hips up high and fold your torso toward your thighs. Draw your thighs away from your kneecaps by engaging your quadriceps. Sink your heels toward the mat. Take 5 full breaths (30 seconds).

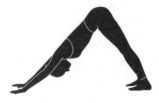

2. **Extended Side Angle Pose:** Inhale, then exhale and move one foot between your hands. Ground your back heel down, bend into your front knee, and twist from your lower torso as you reach your left hand up toward the ceiling. Keep your right hand on the floor next to your foot. Work to stack your shoulders on top of each other and spiral your ribs toward the ceiling. Reach up toward your top hand rather than down toward the ground. Take 5 full breaths (30 seconds). Repeat Extended Side Angle Pose on the other side.

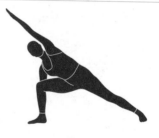

3. **Downward-Facing Dog:** Exhale, plant your hands, and step your feet back behind you. Send your hips up high and fold your torso toward your thighs. Draw your thighs away from your kneecaps by engaging your quadriceps. Sink your heels toward the mat. Take 5 full breaths (30 seconds).

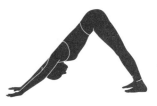

4. **Plank Pose:** Exhale, plant your hands palms down, shoulder-width apart, and extend your legs behind you. Place your feet hip-width apart with your toes pointed down. Create one long line of energy from your heels to the top of your head. Inhale.

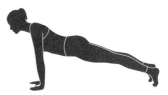

5. **Four-Limbed Staff Pose:** On your next exhale, bend your elbows and lower your entire body halfway to the mat. Keep your elbows close to your sides and make sure your elbows don't bend more than 90 degrees.

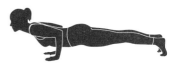

6. **Upward-Facing Dog:** On your next breath in, press down through your palms, straighten your elbows, and open up through your chest. Stack your shoulders

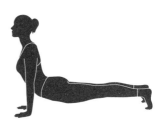

directly over your wrists and engage your legs enough to lift your knees and thighs away from your mat.

7. **Downward-Facing Dog:** Exhale, plant your hands, and step your feet back behind you. Send your hips up high and fold your torso toward your thighs. Draw your thighs away from your kneecaps by engaging your quadriceps. Sink your heels toward the mat. Take 3 full breaths (15 seconds).

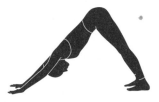

YOGA SEQUENCES FOR STRENGTH

Though you won't use any weights like you'd find in a gym, these sequences will help tone and strengthen nearly every muscle in your body. Just by using your own body weight and a careful application of muscle contractions and releases, you will build strength—both of body and mind.

Strength Sequence 1

1. **Downward-Facing Dog:** Exhale, plant your hands, and step your feet back behind you. Send your hips up high and fold your torso toward your thighs. Draw your thighs away from your kneecaps by engaging your quadriceps. Sink your heels toward the mat. Take 5 full breaths (30 seconds).

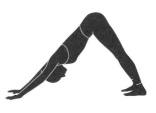

2. **Plank Pose:** Exhale, plant your hands palms down, shoulder-width apart, and extend your legs behind you. Place your feet hip-width apart with your toes pointed down. Create one long line of energy from your heels to the top of your head. Take 20 full breaths (2 minutes). Inhale.

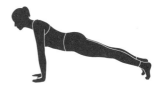

3. **Downward-Facing Dog:** Exhale, plant your hands, and step your feet back behind you. Send your hips up high and fold your torso toward your thighs. Draw your thighs away from your kneecaps by engaging your quadriceps. Sink your heels toward the mat. Take 5 full breaths (30 seconds).

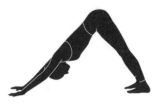

Strength Sequence 2

1. **Downward-Facing Dog:** Exhale, plant your hands, and step your feet back behind you. Send your hips up high and fold your torso toward your thighs. Draw your thighs away from your kneecaps by engaging your quadriceps. Sink your heels toward the mat. Take 5 full breaths (30 seconds).

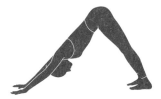

2. **Standing Forward Bend:** Exhale and hinge at your hips. Let your torso drape over your thighs and reach your fingers toward the ground, bending as far as you can comfortably to release your lower back. Take 3 full breaths (15 seconds).

3. **Chair Pose:** Inhale, bend your knees, and sweep your arms up toward the ceiling. Sink your weight into your hips and let the weight sink all the way down into your heels. Squeeze your inner thighs to-gether, keep your lower ribs in, and relax your shoulders away from your ears. Take 10 full breaths (1 minute).

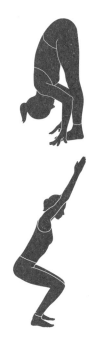

4. **Standing Forward Bend:** Exhale and hinge at your hips. Let your torso drape over your thighs and reach your fingers toward the ground, bending as far as you can comfortably to release your lower back. Take 3 full breaths (15 seconds).

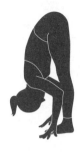

5. **Downward-Facing Dog:** Exhale, plant your hands, and step your feet back behind you. Send your hips up high and fold your torso toward your thighs. Draw your thighs away from your kneecaps by engaging your quadriceps. Sink your heels toward the mat. Take 10 full breaths (1 minute).

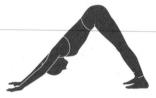

Strength Sequence 3

1. **Downward-Facing Dog:** Exhale, plant your hands, and step your feet back behind you. Send your hips up high and fold your torso toward your thighs. Draw your thighs away from your kneecaps by engaging your quadriceps. Sink your heels toward the mat. Take 5 full breaths (30 seconds).

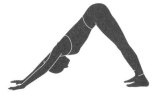

2. **Warrior II:** Inhale as you move into Warrior II—ground your back heel and move your hips to open along with your chest. Lower your arms to extend outward from your shoulders to your fingertips. Bend into your front knee up to 90 degrees and make sure it's stacked directly over your ankle. Keep your back leg engaged and externally rotate your front thigh. Take 10 full breaths (1 minute). Repeat Warrior II on the other side.

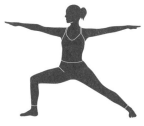

3. **Plank Pose:** Exhale, plant your hands palms down, shoulder-width apart, and extend your legs behind you. Place your feet hip-width apart with your toes pointed down. Create one long line of energy from your heels to the top of your head. Take 10 full breaths (1 minute).

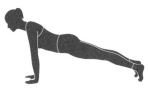

Strength Sequence 4

1. **Downward-Facing Dog:** Exhale, plant your hands, and step your feet back behind you. Send your hips up high and fold your torso toward your thighs. Draw your thighs away from your kneecaps by engaging your quadriceps. Sink your heels toward the mat. Take 5 full breaths (30 seconds).

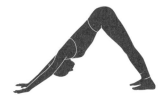

2. **Warrior II:** Inhale as you move into Warrior II—ground your back heel down and move your hips to open along with your chest. Lower your arms to extend outward from your shoulders to your fingertips. Bend into your front knee up to 90 degrees and make sure it's stacked directly over your ankle. Keep your back leg engaged and externally rotate your front thigh. Take 5 full breaths (30 seconds). Repeat Warrior II on the other side.

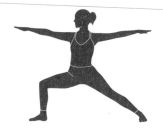

3. **Triangle Pose:** Exhale, keep your feet where they are, straighten your front knee, and twist from your lower torso as you reach your top hand up toward the ceiling and your other hand to the mat. Work to stack your shoulders on top of each other and spiral your ribs toward the ceiling. Reach up toward your top hand rather than down toward the ground. Take 5 full breaths (30 seconds).

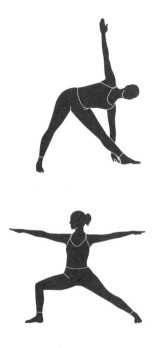

4. **Warrior II:** Inhale as you move into Warrior II—ground your back heel down and move your hips to open along with your chest. Lower your arms to extend outward from your shoulders to your fingertips. Bend into your front knee up to 90 degrees and make sure it's stacked directly over your ankle. Keep your back leg engaged and externally rotate your front thigh. Take 3 full breaths (15 seconds). Repeat Warrior II on the other side.

Strength Sequence 5

1. **Downward-Facing Dog:** Exhale, plant your hands, and step your feet back behind you. Send your hips up high and fold your torso toward your thighs. Draw your thighs away from your kneecaps by engaging your quadriceps. Sink your heels toward the mat. Take 5 full breaths (30 seconds).

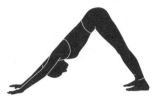

2. **Warrior I:** Inhale, then exhale and move one foot between your hands. Inhale into the position—ground your back heel down, bend your front knee into a 90-degree angle, stack your shoulders over your hips, and reach your arms straight up to the ceiling. Square your hips by drawing your front leg's outer hip back and pressing your opposite hip forward. Take 5 full breaths (30 seconds). Repeat Warrior I on the other side.

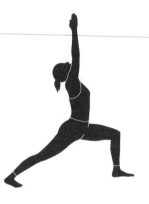

3. **Plank Pose:** Exhale, plant your hands palms down, shoulder-width apart, and extend your legs behind you. Place your feet hip-width apart with your toes

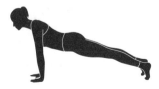

pointed down. Create one long line of energy from your heels to the top of your head. Take 10 full breaths (1 minute).

4. **Downward-Facing Dog:** Exhale, plant your hands, and step your feet back behind you. Send your hips up high and fold your torso toward your thighs. Draw your thighs away from your kneecaps by engaging your quadriceps. Sink your heels toward the mat. Take 5 full breaths (30 seconds).

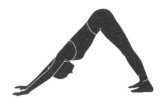

Strength Sequence 6

1. **Downward-Facing Dog:** Exhale, plant your hands, and step your feet back behind you. Send your hips up high and fold your torso toward your thighs. Draw your thighs away from your kneecaps by engaging your quadriceps. Sink your heels toward the mat. Take 5 full breaths (30 seconds).

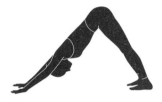

2. **Plank Pose:** Exhale, plant your hands palms down, shoulder-width apart, and extend your legs behind you. Place your feet hip-width apart with your toes pointed down. Create one long line of energy from your heels to the top of your head. Take 10 full breaths (1 minute). Inhale.

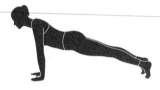

3. **Cobra:** Exhale, lower down to your belly, bring your hands directly underneath your shoulders by your lower ribs, and bring your legs together. On an inhale, peel your chest away from the mat using your body and putting little to no weight on your hands. Straighten out your legs and stretch your chest forward with your hands palms

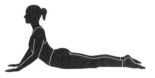

down, arms lightly bent at the elbow, and your chest and head aligned. Take 5 full breaths (30 seconds).

4. **Plank Pose:** Exhale, plant your hands palms down, shoulder-width apart, and extend your legs behind you. Place your feet hip-width apart with your toes pointed down. Create one long line of energy from your heels to the top of your head. Take 10 full breaths (1 minute).

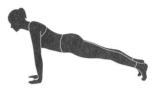

5. **Downward-Facing Dog:** Exhale, plant your hands, and step your feet back behind you. Send your hips up high and fold your torso toward your thighs. Draw your thighs away from your kneecaps by engaging your quadriceps. Sink your heels toward the mat. Take 5 full breaths (30 seconds).

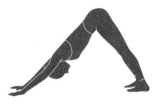

Strength Sequence 7

1. **Downward-Facing Dog:** Exhale, plant your hands, and step your feet back behind you. Send your hips up high and fold your torso toward your thighs. Draw your thighs away from your kneecaps by engaging your quadriceps. Sink your heels toward the mat. Take 5 full breaths (30 seconds).

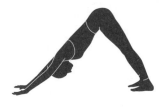

2. **Plank Pose:** Exhale, plant your hands palms down, shoulder-width apart, and extend your legs behind you. Place your feet hip-width apart with your toes pointed down. Create one long line of energy from your heels to the top of your head. Take 10 full breaths (1 minute). Inhale.

3. **Four-Limbed Staff Pose:** On your next exhale, bend your elbows and lower your entire body halfway to the mat. Keep your elbows close to your sides and make sure your elbows don't bend more than 90 degrees.

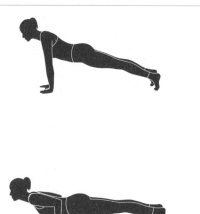

4. **Plank Pose:** Inhale and press into your palms to slowly lift your body by straightening your arms. Create one long line of energy from your heels to the top of your head. Take 10 breaths (1 minute).

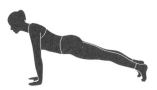

5. **Downward-Facing Dog:** Exhale, plant your hands, and step your feet back behind you. Send your hips up high and fold your torso toward your thighs. Draw your thighs away from your kneecaps by engaging your quadriceps. Sink your heels toward the mat. Take 5 full breaths (30 seconds).

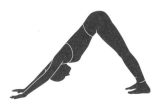

Strength Sequence 8

1. **Downward-Facing Dog:** Exhale, plant your hands, and step your feet back behind you. Send your hips up high and fold your torso toward your thighs. Draw your thighs away from your kneecaps by engaging your quadriceps. Sink your heels toward the mat. Take 5 full breaths (30 seconds).

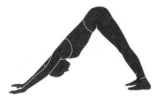

2. **Plank Pose:** Exhale, plant your hands palms down, shoulder-width apart, and extend your legs behind you. Place your feet hip-width apart with your toes pointed down. Create one long line of energy from your heels to the top of your head. Take 10 full breaths (1 minute).

3. **Four-Limbed Staff Pose:** On your next exhale, bend your elbows and lower your entire body halfway to the mat. Keep your elbows close to your sides and make sure your elbows don't bend more than 90 degrees.

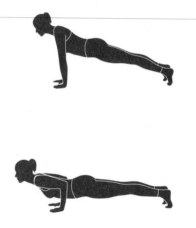

4. **Upward-Facing Dog:** On your next inhale, press down through your palms, straighten your elbows, and open up through your chest. Stack your shoulders directly over your wrists and engage your legs enough to lift your knees and thighs away from your mat.

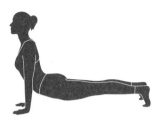

5. **Downward-Facing Dog:** Exhale, plant your hands, and step your feet back behind you. Send your hips up high and fold your torso toward your thighs. Draw your thighs away from your kneecaps by engaging your quadriceps. Sink your heels toward the mat. Take 5 full breaths (30 seconds).

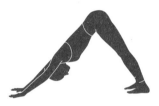

Strength Sequence 9

1. **Downward-Facing Dog:** Exhale, plant your hands, and step your feet back behind you. Send your hips up high and fold your torso toward your thighs. Draw your thighs away from your kneecaps by engaging your quadriceps. Sink your heels toward the mat. Take 5 full breaths (30 seconds).

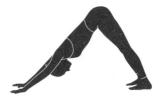

2. **Plank Pose:** Exhale, plant your hands palms down, shoulder-width apart, and extend your legs behind you. Place your feet hip-width apart with your toes pointed down. Create one long line of energy from your heels to the top of your head. Take 10 full breaths (1 minute).

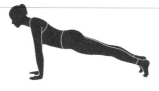

3. **Cobra Pose:** Exhale, lower down to your belly, bring your hands directly underneath your shoulders by your lower ribs, and bring your legs together. On an inhale, peel your chest away from the mat using your body and putting little to no weight on your hands. Straighten out your legs and stretch your chest forward with

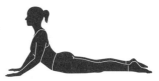

your hands palms down, arms lightly bent at the elbow, and your chest and head aligned. Take 5 full breaths (30 seconds).

4. **Locust Pose:** Extend your arms above your head with your palms facing each other. Inhale and lift your arms, legs, and chest off your mat; as you exhale, roll onto the soft part of your belly. Squeeze your inner thighs together and keep your gaze down to protect your neck. Engage your muscles to lift as high as you can while continuing to breathe. Take 5 full breaths (30 seconds).

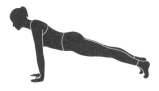

5. **Plank Pose:** Exhale, plant your hands palms down, shoulder-width apart, and extend your legs behind you. Place your feet hip-width apart with your toes pointed down. Create one long line of energy from your heels to the top of your head. Take 10 full breaths (1 minute).

6. **Downward-Facing Dog:** Exhale, plant your hands, and step your feet back behind you. Send your hips up high and fold your torso toward your thighs. Draw your thighs away from your kneecaps by engaging your quadriceps. Sink your heels toward the mat. Take 5 full breaths (30 seconds).

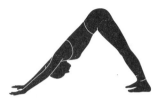

Strength Sequence 10

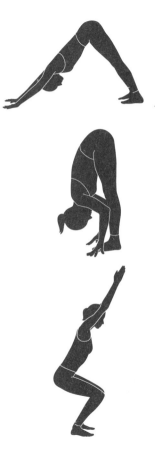

1. **Downward-Facing Dog:** Exhale, plant your hands, and step your feet back behind you. Send your hips up high and fold your torso toward your thighs. Draw your thighs away from your kneecaps by engaging your quadriceps. Sink your heels toward the mat. Take 5 full breaths (30 seconds).

2. **Standing Forward Bend:** Exhale and hinge at your hips. Let your torso drape over your thighs and reach your fingers toward the ground, bending as far as you can comfortably to release your lower back. Take 3 full breaths (15 seconds).

3. **Chair Pose:** Inhale, bend your knees, and sweep your arms up toward the ceiling. Sink your weight into your hips and let the weight sink all the way down into your heels. Squeeze your inner thighs together, keep your lower ribs in, and relax your shoulders away from your ears. Take 10 full breaths (1 minute).

4. **Mountain Pose:** Stand tall, inhale, and reach your arms straight up to the ceiling. Ground down through the soles of your feet and squeeze your inner thighs together. Keep your lower ribs in and turn your pinkies inward to relax your shoulders away from your ears. Take 3 full breaths (15 seconds). Return your arms to your sides.

5. **Chair Pose:** Inhale, bend your knees, and sweep your arms up toward the ceiling. Sink your weight into your hips and let the weight sink all the way down into your heels. Squeeze your inner thighs together, keep your lower ribs in, and relax your shoulders away from your ears. Take 5 full breaths (30 seconds).

6. **Standing Forward Bend:** Exhale and hinge at your hips. Let your torso drape over your thighs and reach your fingers toward the ground, bending as far as you can comfortably to release your lower back. Take 3 full breaths (15 seconds).

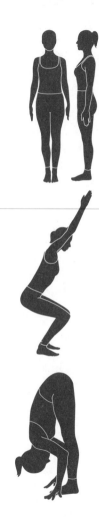

7. **Downward-Facing Dog:** Exhale, plant your hands, and step your feet back behind you. Send your hips up high and fold your torso toward your thighs. Draw your thighs away from your kneecaps by engaging your quadriceps. Sink your heels toward the mat. Take 5 full breaths (30 seconds).

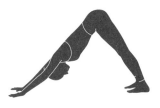

YOGA SEQUENCES FOR FLEXIBILITY

Some people think of yoga practice as twisting yourself into limb-bending pretzel-like shapes on a mountaintop in the middle of nowhere. Though that's far from the truth, doing yoga regularly will indeed improve your flexibility in safe and simple ways. These sequences will have you reaching farther than you imagined you could, from head to toe.

Flexibility Sequence 1

1. **Easy Pose:** Sit up tall on one or two folded blankets with your legs crossed. Rest your hands on the mat beside your hips or bring your palms to prayer at your heart center and close your eyes. Take 10 full breaths (1 minute).

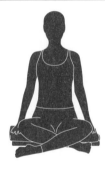

2. **Seated Straight-Leg Forward Bend:** Sit with your legs extended in front of you. Inhale to lengthen your spine, exhale, then hinge at your hips and reach for your toes, keeping your back flat. Clasp your hands together with your palms out, leaning forward as far as you can. Take 20 full breaths (2 minutes).

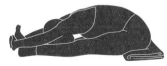

3. **Basic Relaxation Pose:** Lie flat on your mat and extend your arms and legs. With your palms facing up, surrender to all effort and allow your body to melt into your mat. Let your muscles relax completely and allow all tension to drip off your fingertips and toes. Relax and breathe for 2 minutes.

Flexibility Sequence 2

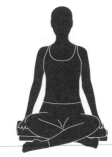

1. **Easy Pose:** Sit up tall on one or two folded blankets with your legs crossed. Rest your hands on the mat beside your hips or bring your palms to prayer at your heart center and close your eyes. Take 10 full breaths (1 minute).

2. **Belly Twist:** Lie on your back and as you inhale, draw your knees into your chest. As you exhale, let your legs drop over to your left side, keeping your legs together and bent and your torso and arms flat on the mat. Twist your hips so your legs rest flat on the mat with your knees stacked on top of each other. Extend your arms out to the right and left in line with your shoulders and send your gaze over to the left for the full expression of this twist. Take 10 full breaths (1 minute). Repeat Belly Twist on the other side.

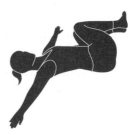

3. **Basic Relaxation Pose:** Extend your arms and legs flat on your mat. With your palms facing up, surrender to all effort and allow your body to melt into your mat. Let your muscles relax completely and allow all tension to drip off your fingertips and toes. Relax and breathe for 2 minutes.

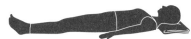

Flexibility Sequence 3

1. **Easy Pose:** Sit up tall on one or two folded blankets with your legs crossed. Rest your hands on the mat beside your hips or bring your palms to prayer at your heart center and close your eyes. Take 20 full breaths (2 minutes).

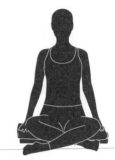

2. **Reclining Hand-to-Big-Toe Pose I:** Lie on your back and bring your knees into your chest. Grab your right big toe with your index and middle finger (or wrap a strap around the ball of your foot) and straighten out your leg in front of you as far as you can. Extend your left leg and keep your shoulders and head flat on the mat. Take 10 full breaths (1 minute). Repeat Reclining Hand-to-Big-Toe Pose I on the other side.

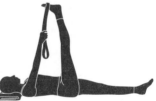

3. **Basic Relaxation Pose:** Extend your arms and legs flat on your mat. With your palms facing up, surrender to all effort and allow your body to melt into your mat. Let your muscles relax completely and allow all tension to drip off your fingertips and toes. Relax and breathe for 1 minute.

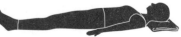

Flexibility Sequence 4

1. **Reclining Hand-to-Big-Toe Pose I:** Lie on your back and bring your knees into your chest. Grab your right big toe with your index and middle finger (or wrap a strap around the ball of your foot) and straighten out your leg in front of you as far as you can. Extend your left leg and keep your shoulders and head flat on the mat. Take 5 full breaths (30 seconds).

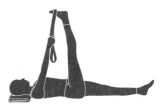

2. **Reclining Hand-to-Big-Toe Pose II:** Send your leg over to the side of your body and work to straighten the arm that is holding your toe. Take 5 full breaths (30 seconds). Repeat Reclining Hand-to-Big-Toe Pose I and II on the other side.

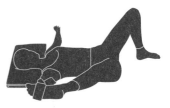

3. **Basic Relaxation Pose:** Extend your arms and legs flat on your mat. With your palms facing up, surrender to all effort and allow your body to melt into your mat. Let your muscles relax completely and allow all tension to drip off your fingertips and toes. Relax and breathe for 1 minute.

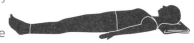

Flexibility Sequence 5

1. **Bridge Pose:** Lie down on your back, bend your knees, and place your feet a bit more than hip-width apart, flat on the mat. Inhale as you raise your hips. Exhale, shimmy your shoulders underneath you, and extend your arms, clenching your hands into fists. Breathe air into your belly and find space across your chest. Take 10 full breaths (1 minute).

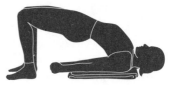

2. **Supported Bound Angle Pose:** Lie on your back and bend your knees (place folded blankets or bolsters under your head, back, and knees, if you prefer). Bring the soles of your feet together to touch and allow your knees to splay out to the sides. Close your eyes and extend your arms out to your sides as you breathe. Take 20 full breaths (2 minutes).

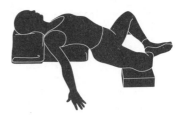

3. **Basic Relaxation Pose:** Extend your arms and legs flat on your mat. With your palms facing up, surrender to all effort and allow your body to melt into your mat. Let your muscles relax completely and allow all tension to drip off your fingertips and toes. Relax and breathe for 2 minutes.

Flexibility Sequence 6

1. **Downward-Facing Dog:** Exhale, plant your hands, and step your feet back behind you. Send your hips up high and fold your torso toward your thighs. Draw your thighs away from your kneecaps by engaging your quadriceps. Sink your heels toward the mat. Take 10 full breaths (1 minute).

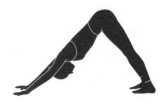

2. **Intense Side Stretch Pose:** Exhale, jump or walk your feet wide apart, and hinge at your hips, leaning down toward your front leg. Keep your back and neck straight and lead with your chest. Fold your arms behind your back. Take 10 full breaths (1 minute). Repeat Intense Side Stretch Pose on the other side.

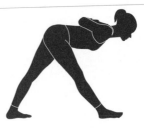

3. **Downward-Facing Dog:** Exhale, plant your hands, and step your feet back behind you. Send your hips up high and fold your torso toward your thighs. Draw your thighs away from your kneecaps by engaging your quadriceps. Sink your heels toward the mat. Take 20 full breaths (2 minutes).

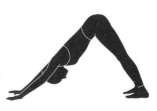

Flexibility Sequence 7

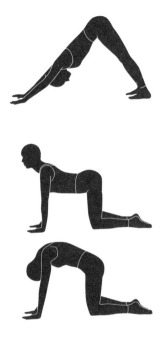

1. **Downward-Facing Dog:** Exhale, plant your hands, and step your feet back behind you. Send your hips up high and fold your torso toward your thighs. Draw your thighs away from your kneecaps by engaging your quadriceps. Sink your heels toward the mat. Take 10 full breaths (1 minute).

2. **Cat-Cow:** Exhale and drop down to your hands and knees. Inhale, drop your belly, and arch your back, raising your tailbone. Lift your gaze as you find expansion across your chest. Exhale, arch your spine up, and lower your tailbone. Let your head hang heavy and look down between your thighs. Take 20 full breaths (2 minutes).

3. **Basic Relaxation Pose:** Lie flat on your mat and extend your arms and legs. With your palms facing up, surrender to all effort and allow your body to melt into your mat. Let your muscles relax completely and allow all tension to drip off your fingertips and toes. Relax and breathe for 2 minutes.

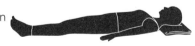

Flexibility Sequence 8

1. **Downward-Facing Dog:** Exhale, plant your hands, and step your feet back behind you. Send your hips up high and fold your torso toward your thighs. Draw your thighs away from your kneecaps by engaging your quadriceps. Sink your heels toward the mat. Take 5 full breaths (30 seconds).

2. **Cat-Cow:** Exhale and drop down to your hands and knees. Inhale, drop your belly, and arch your back, raising your tailbone. Lift your gaze as you find expansion across your chest. Exhale, arch your spine up, and lower your tailbone. Let your head hang heavy and look down between your thighs. Take 10 full breaths (1 minute).

3. **Pigeon Pose:** Bring your right leg in front of you, bent at the knee, and extend your left leg straight behind you with the top of your foot flat on your mat. Square your hips the best you can and then draw your chest forward as you walk your hands out in front of you, keeping your back straight. Take 10 full breaths (1 minute). Repeat Pigeon Pose on the other side.

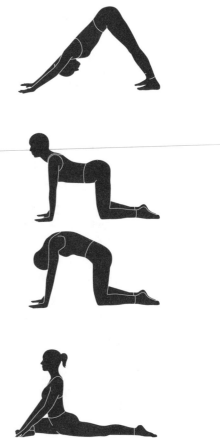

Flexibility Sequence 9

1. **Downward-Facing Dog:** Exhale, plant your
   hands, and step your feet back behind
   you. Send your hips up high and fold your
   torso toward your thighs. Draw your thighs
   away from your kneecaps by engaging your
   quadriceps. Sink your heels toward the mat.
   Take 5 full breaths (30 seconds).

2. **Cat-Cow:** Exhale and drop down to your
   hands and knees. Inhale, drop your belly,
   and arch your back, raising your tailbone.
   Lift your gaze as you find expansion
   across your chest. Exhale, arch your spine
   up, and lower your tailbone. Let your head
   hang heavy and look down between your
   thighs. Take 10 full breaths as you move
   through this pose (1 minute).

3. **Equestrian Pose:** Inhale, then exhale and
   place your left foot between your hands.
   Inhale into the pose—drop down to your
   left knee and bring your fingertips to the
   floor directly under your shoulders. Work
   to stack your shoulders directly on top of
   your hips and open your chest. Take 10 full

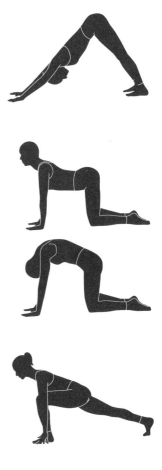

breaths (1 minute). Repeat Equestrian
Pose on the other side.

4. **Basic Relaxation Pose:** Lie flat on your
   mat and extend your arms and legs.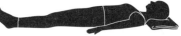
   With your palms facing up, surrender
   to all effort and allow your body to
   melt into your mat. Let your muscles relax
   completely and allow all tension to drip
   off your fingertips and toes. Relax and
   breathe for 1 minute.

Flexibility Sequence 10

1. **Downward-Facing Dog:** Exhale, plant your hands, and step your feet back behind you. Send your hips up high and fold your torso toward your thighs. Draw your thighs away from your kneecaps by engaging your quadriceps. Sink your heels toward the mat. Take 5 full breaths (30 seconds).

2. **Cat-Cow:** Exhale and drop down to your hands and knees. Inhale, drop your belly, and arch your back, raising your tailbone. Lift your gaze as you find expansion across your chest. Exhale, arch your spine up, and lower your tailbone. Let your head hang heavy and look down between your thighs. Take 10 full breaths (1 minute).

3. **Supported Bound Angle Pose:** Lie on your back and bend your knees (place folded blankets or bolsters under your head, back, and knees, if you prefer). Bring the soles of your feet together to touch and allow your knees to splay

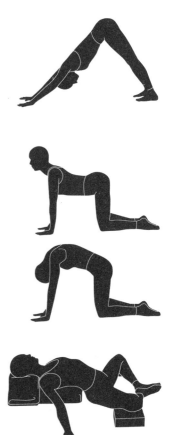

out to the sides. Close your eyes and extend your arms out to your sides as you breathe. Take 10 full breaths (1 minute).

4. **Basic Relaxation Pose:** Extend your arms and legs flat on your mat. With your palms facing up, surrender to all effort and allow your body to melt into your mat. Let your muscles relax completely and allow all tension to drip off your fingertips and toes. Relax and breathe for 2 minutes.

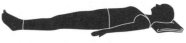

YOGA SEQUENCES FOR WEIGHT LOSS

Many aspects of health contribute to overall weight loss, and yoga is a perfect way to incorporate exercise and mindfulness into your plan. When you quiet your mind and focus on what's important, you can put your body's needs first. Whether your plan includes healthy foods, adequate sleep, or calorie-burning exercise, these yoga sequences will complement your efforts.

Weight Loss Sequence 1

1. **Plank Pose:** Exhale, plant your hands palms down, shoulder-width apart, and extend your legs behind you. Place your feet hip-width apart with your toes pointed down. Create one long line of energy from your heels to the top of your head. Take 10 full breaths (1 minute).

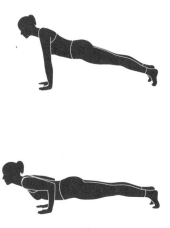

2. **Four-Limbed Staff Pose:** On your next exhale, bend your elbows and lower your entire body halfway to the mat. Keep your elbows close to your sides and make sure your elbows don't bend more than 90 degrees.

3. **Plank Pose:** Inhale and press into your palms to slowly lift your body by straightening your arms. Create one long line of energy from your heels to the top of your head. Take 5 full breaths (30 seconds).

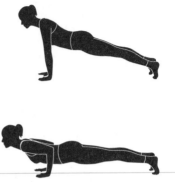

4. **Four-Limbed Staff Pose:** On your next exhale, bend your elbows and lower your entire body halfway to the mat. Keep your elbows close to your sides and make sure your elbows don't bend more than 90 degrees.

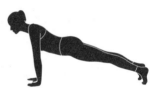

5. **Plank Pose:** Inhale and press into your palms to slowly lift your body by straightening your arms. Create one long line of energy from your heels to the top of your head. Take 3 full breaths (15 seconds).

6. **Downward-Facing Dog:** Exhale, plant your hands, and step your feet back behind you. Send your hips up high and fold your torso toward your thighs. Draw your thighs away from your kneecaps by engaging your quadriceps. Sink your heels toward the mat. Take 5 full breaths (30 seconds).

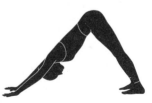

Weight Loss Sequence 2

1. **Plank Pose:** Exhale, plant your hands palms down, shoulder-width apart, and extend your legs behind you. Place your feet hip-width apart with your toes pointed down. Create one long line of energy from your heels to the top of your head. Take 10 full breaths (1 minute).

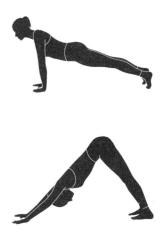

2. **Downward-Facing Dog:** Exhale, plant your hands, and step your feet back behind you. Send your hips up high and fold your torso toward your thighs. Draw your thighs away from your knee-caps by engaging your quadriceps. Sink your heels toward the mat. Take 5 full breaths (30 seconds).

3. **Standing Forward Bend:** Exhale and hinge at your hips. Let your torso drape over your thighs and reach your fingers toward the ground, bending as far as you can comfortably to release your lower back. Take 5 full breaths (30 seconds).

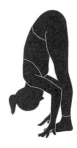

4. **Chair Pose:** Inhale, bend your knees, and sweep your arms up toward the ceiling. Sink your weight into your hips and let the weight sink all the way down into your heels. Squeeze your inner thighs together, keep your lower ribs in, and relax your shoulders away from your ears. Take 5 full breaths (30 seconds).

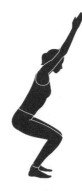

5. **Standing Forward Bend:** Exhale and hinge at your hips. Let your torso drape over your thighs and reach your fingers toward the ground, bending as far as you can comfortably to release your lower back. Take 5 full breaths (30 seconds).

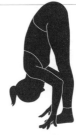

6. **Downward-Facing Dog:** Exhale, plant your hands, and step your feet back behind you. Send your hips up high and fold your torso toward your thighs. Draw your thighs away from your knee-caps by engaging your quadriceps. Sink your heels toward the mat. Take 10 full breaths (1 minute).

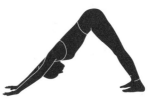

Weight Loss Sequence 3

1. **Plank Pose:** Exhale, plant your hands palms down, shoulder-width apart, and extend your legs behind you. Place your feet hip-width apart with your toes pointed down. Create one long line of energy from your heels to the top of your head. Take 5 full breaths (30 seconds).

2. **Downward-Facing Dog:** Exhale, plant your hands, and step your feet back behind you. Send your hips up high and fold your torso toward your thighs. Draw your thighs away from your kneecaps by engaging your quadriceps. Sink your heels toward the mat. Take 5 full breaths (30 seconds).

3. **Warrior I:** Inhale, then exhale and move one foot between your hands. Inhale into the position—ground your back heel down, bend your front knee into a 90-degree angle, stack your shoulders over your hips, and reach your arms straight up to the ceiling. Square your hips by drawing your front leg's outer hip back and pressing your opposite hip forward.

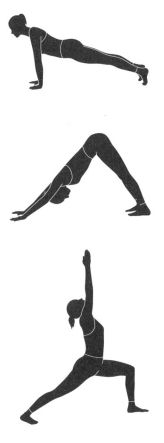

Take 5 full breaths (30 seconds). Repeat
Warrior I on the other side.

4. **Warrior II:** Inhale as you move into Warrior II—ground your back heel down and
move your hips to open along with your
chest. Lower your arms to extend outward
from your shoulders to your fingertips.
Bend into your front knee up to 90 degrees and make sure it's stacked directly
over your ankle. Keep your back leg engaged and externally rotate your front
thigh. Take 5 full breaths (30 seconds).
Repeat Warrior II on the other side.

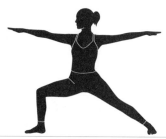

5. **Downward-Facing Dog:** Exhale, plant your
hands, and step your feet back behind
you. Send your hips up high and fold your
torso toward your thighs. Draw your thighs
away from your kneecaps by engaging your
quadriceps. Sink your heels toward the
mat. Take 5 full breaths (30 seconds).

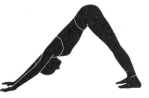

Weight Loss Sequence 4

1. **Plank Pose:** Exhale, plant your hands palms down, shoulder-width apart, and extend your legs behind you. Place your feet hip-width apart with your toes pointed down. Create one long line of energy from your heels to the top of your head. Take 5 full breaths (30 seconds).

2. **Equestrian Pose:** Inhale, then exhale and place your left foot between your hands. Inhale into the pose—drop down to your left knee and bring your fingertips to the floor directly under your shoulders. Work to stack your shoulders directly on top of your hips and open your chest. Take 5 full breaths (30 seconds). Repeat Equestrian Pose on the other side.

3. **Standing Forward Bend:** Exhale and hinge at your hips. Let your torso drape over your thighs and reach your fingers toward the ground, bending as far as you can comfortably to release your lower back. Take 5 full breaths (30 seconds).

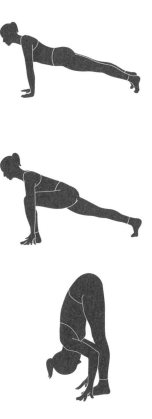

4. **Plank Pose:** Exhale, plant your hands palms down, shoulder-width apart, and extend your legs behind you. Place your feet hip-width apart with your toes pointed down. Create one long line of energy from your heels to the top of your head. Take 10 full breaths (1 minute).

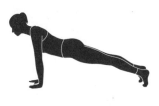

5. **Downward-Facing Dog:** Exhale, plant your hands, and step your feet back behind you. Send your hips up high and fold your torso toward your thighs. Draw your thighs away from your kneecaps by engaging your quadriceps. Sink your heels toward the mat. Take 5 full breaths (30 seconds).

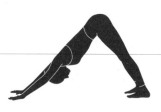

Weight Loss Sequence 5

1. **Plank Pose:** Exhale, plant your hands palms down, shoulder-width apart, and extend your legs behind you. Place your feet hip-width apart with your toes pointed down. Create one long line of energy from your heels to the top of your head. Take 5 full breaths (30 seconds).

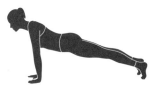

2. **Cobra Pose:** Exhale, lower down to your belly, bring your hands directly underneath your shoulders by your lower ribs, and bring your legs together. On an inhale, peel your chest away from the mat using your body and putting little to no weight on your hands. Straighten out your legs and stretch your chest forward with your hands palms down, arms lightly bent at the elbow, and your chest and head aligned. Take 5 full breaths (30 seconds).

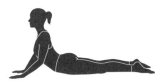

3. **Locust Pose:** Extend your arms above your head with your palms facing each other. Inhale and lift your arms, legs, and chest off your

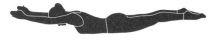

mat; as you exhale, roll onto the soft part of your belly. Squeeze your inner thighs together and keep your gaze down to protect your neck. Engage your muscles to lift as high as you can while continuing to breathe. Take 5 full breaths (30 seconds).

4. **Plank Pose:** Exhale, plant your hands palms down, shoulder-width apart, and extend your legs behind you. Place your feet hip-width apart with your toes pointed down. Create one long line of energy from your heels to the top of your head. Take 10 full breaths (1 minute).

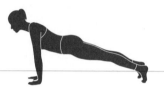

5. **Downward-Facing Dog:** Exhale, plant your hands, and step your feet back behind you. Send your hips up high and fold your torso toward your thighs. Draw your thighs away from your kneecaps by engaging your quadriceps. Sink your heels toward the mat. Take 5 full breaths (30 seconds).

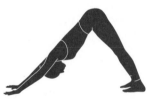

Weight Loss Sequence 6

1. **Plank Pose:** Exhale, plant your hands palms down, shoulder-width apart, and extend your legs behind you. Place your feet hip-width apart with your toes pointed down. Create one long line of energy from your heels to the top of your head. Take 5 full breaths (30 seconds).

2. **Standing Forward Bend:** Exhale and hinge at your hips. Let your torso drape over your thighs and reach your fingers toward the ground, bending as far as you can comfortably to release your lower back. Take 5 full breaths (30 seconds).

3. **Standing Half-Forward Bend:** For one breath in, place your hands on the chair in front of you and breathe. Create one line of energy from your tailbone to the top of your head. Engage your shoulder blades together and down your back. Take 5 full breaths (30 seconds).

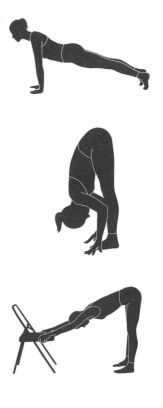

4. **Plank Pose:** Exhale, plant your hands palms down, shoulder-width apart, and extend your legs behind you. Place your feet hip-width apart with your toes pointed down. Create one long line of energy from your heels to the top of your head. Take 10 full breaths (1 minute). Inhale.

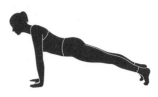

5. **Four-Limbed Staff Pose:** On your next exhale, bend your elbows and lower your entire body halfway to the mat. Keep your elbows close to your sides and make sure your elbows don't bend more than 90 degrees.

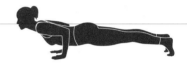

6. **Upward-Facing Dog:** For your next breath in, press down through your palms, straighten your elbows, and open up through your chest. Stack your shoulders directly over your wrists and engage your legs enough to lift your knees and thighs away from your mat.

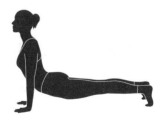

7. **Downward-Facing Dog:** Exhale, plant your hands, and step your feet back behind you. Send your hips up high and fold your torso toward your thighs. Draw your thighs away from your kneecaps by engaging your quadriceps. Sink your heels toward the mat. Take 5 full breaths (30 seconds).

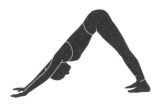

Weight Loss Sequence 7

1. **Plank Pose:** Exhale, plant your hands palms down, shoulder-width apart, and extend your legs behind you. Place your feet hip-width apart with your toes pointed down. Create one long line of energy from your heels to the top of your head. Take 5 full breaths (30 seconds).

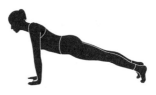

2. **Extended Side Angle Pose:** Inhale, then exhale and move one foot between your hands. Ground your back heel down, bend into your front knee, and twist from your lower torso as you reach your left hand up toward the ceiling. Keep your right hand on the floor next to your foot. Work to stack your shoulders on top of each other and spiral your ribs toward the ceiling. Reach up toward your top hand rather than down toward the ground. Take 5 full breaths (30 seconds). Repeat Extended Side Angle Pose on the other side.

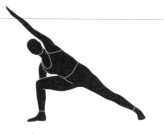

3. **Plank Pose:** Exhale, plant your hands palms down, shoulder-width apart, and extend your legs behind you. Place your feet hip-width apart with your toes pointed down. Create one long line of energy from your heels to the top of your head. Take 5 full breaths (30 seconds).

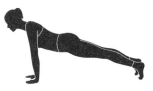

4. **Four-Limbed Staff Pose:** On your next exhale, bend your elbows and lower your entire body halfway to the mat. Keep your elbows close to your sides and make sure your elbows don't bend more than 90 degrees.

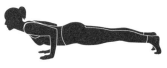

5. **Plank Pose:** Inhale and press into your palms to slowly lift your body by straightening your arms. Create one long line of energy from your heels to the top of your head. Take 5 full breaths (30 seconds).

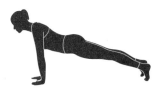

Weight Loss Sequence 8

1. **Plank Pose:** Exhale, plant your hands palms down, shoulder-width apart, and extend your legs behind you. Place your feet hip-width apart with your toes pointed down. Create one long line of energy from your heels to the top of your head. Take 5 full breaths (30 seconds).

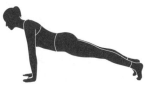

2. **Warrior II:** Inhale as you move into Warrior II—ground your back heel down and move your hips to open along with your chest. Lower your arms to extend outward from your shoulders to your fingertips. Bend into your front knee up to 90 degrees and make sure it's stacked directly over your ankle. Keep your back leg engaged and externally rotate your front thigh. Take 5 full breaths (30 seconds). Repeat Warrior II on the other side.

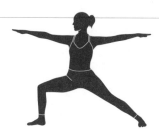

3. **Plank Pose:** Exhale, plant your hands palms down, shoulder-width apart, and extend your legs behind you. Place your feet hip-width apart with your toes

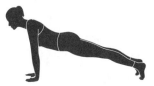

pointed down. Create one long line of energy from your heels to the top of your head. Take 10 full breaths (1 minute).

4. **Four-Limbed Staff Pose:** On your next exhale, bend your elbows and lower your entire body halfway to the mat. Keep your elbows close to your sides and make sure your elbows don't bend more than 90 degrees.

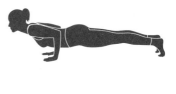

5. **Plank Pose:** Inhale and press into your palms to slowly lift your body by straightening your arms. Create one long line of energy from your heels to the top of your head. Take 5 full breaths (30 seconds).

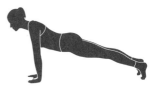

Weight Loss Sequence 9

1. **Plank Pose:** Exhale, plant your hands palms down, shoulder-width apart, and extend your legs behind you. Place your feet hip-width apart with your toes pointed down. Create one long line of energy from your heels to the top of your head. Take 5 full breaths (30 seconds).

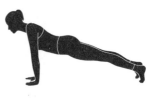

2. **Warrior II:** Inhale as you move into Warrior II—ground your back heel down and move your hips to open along with your chest. Lower your arms to extend outward from your shoulders to your fingertips. Bend into your front knee up to 90 degrees and make sure it's stacked directly over your ankle. Keep your back leg engaged and externally rotate your front thigh. Take 5 full breaths (30 seconds). Repeat Warrior II on the other side.

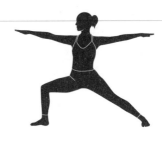

3. **Extended Side Angle Pose:** Inhale, then exhale and move one foot between your hands. Ground your back heel down, bend into your front knee, and twist from your lower torso as you reach your left hand up

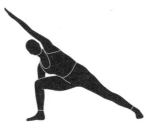

toward the ceiling. Keep your right hand on the floor next to your foot. Work to stack your shoulders on top of each other and spiral your ribs toward the ceiling. Reach up toward your top hand rather than down toward the ground. Take 5 full breaths (30 seconds). Repeat Extended Side Angle Pose on the other side.

4. **Warrior II:** Inhale as you move into Warrior II—ground your back heel down and move your hips to open along with your chest. Lower your arms to extend outward from your shoulders to your fingertips. Bend into your front knee up to 90 degrees and make sure it's stacked directly over your ankle. Keep your back leg engaged and externally rotate your front thigh. Take 5 full breaths (30 seconds). Repeat Warrior II on the other side.

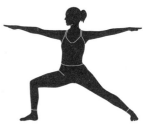

5. **Plank Pose:** Exhale, plant your hands palms down, shoulder-width apart, and extend your legs behind you. Place your feet hip-width apart with your toes pointed down. Create one long line of energy from your heels to the top of your head. Take 5 full breaths (30 seconds).

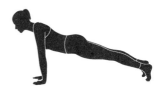

Weight Loss Sequence 10

1. **Plank Pose:** Exhale, plant your hands palms down, shoulder-width apart, and extend your legs behind you. Place your feet hip-width apart with your toes pointed down. Create one long line of energy from your heels to the top of your head. Take 5 full breaths (30 seconds).

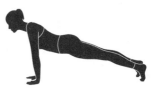

2. **Triangle Pose:** Stand tall and walk your feet apart as far as you can comfortably. Turn your right foot in and rotate your left foot out, keeping your heels in line with each other. Exhale and extend laterally over your left leg, bending from the hip. Lower your left arm and place your fingertips lightly on your left shin or on the floor. Raise your right arm straight up, stacking your shoulders. Look straight ahead. Take 5 full breaths (30 seconds). Repeat Triangle Pose on the other side.

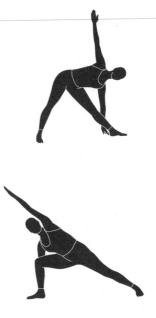

3. **Extended Side Angle Pose:** Inhale, then exhale and move one foot between your hands. Ground your back heel down, bend into your front knee, and twist from

your lower torso as you reach your left hand up toward the ceiling. Keep your right hand on the floor next to your foot. Work to stack your shoulders on top of each other and spiral your ribs toward the ceiling. Reach up toward your top hand rather than down toward the ground. Take 5 full breaths (30 seconds). Repeat Extended Side Angle Pose on the other side.

4. **Triangle Pose:** Inhale, straighten your front knee, and twist from your lower torso as you reach your top hand up toward the ceiling. Work to stack your shoulders on top of each other and spiral your ribs toward the ceiling. Reach up toward your top hand rather than down toward the ground. Take 5 full breaths (30 seconds).

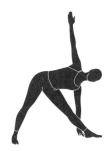

GLOSSARY OF
POSES

Basic Relaxation Pose (Savasana)

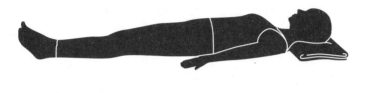

- Lie down on your back with your arms and legs extended. Use a folded blanket under your head and neck so your forehead and chin are level with each other. Turn your palms up while rotating your upper arms outward. Place your arms slightly away from the sides of your body.
- Balance the sides of your body, arms, and legs, feeling equal weight on your shoulders, buttocks, arms, and legs. Then release the effort. Soften your entire body.
- Deepen your next exhalation and lengthen the following inhalation. Move your fingers and toes, and stretch your arms above your head. Bend your knees, slowly roll onto your right side, and use your hands and arms to come to a seated position.

Belly Twist (Jathara Parivartanasana)

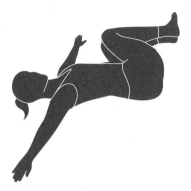

- Lie down and bend your knees with your feet flat on the floor. Lift your feet away from the floor and bring your knees to your chest.
- Extend your arms horizontally on the floor. Stack your knees and ankles and let your knees come down to the floor on the left side at 90 degrees. Gaze up at the ceiling.
- Maintain the length of your spine upon inhalation, twist on exhalation, and roll your right shoulder down toward the floor (without forcing). Stay in the pose for several breaths, deepening the twist. Then bring your knees back to your chest and repeat on the other side.

Bound Angle Pose (Baddha Konasana)

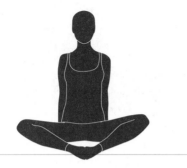

- Sit evenly on your buttocks. Bring the soles of your feet together in front of you and let your knees drop out to the sides.
- Using your hands, draw your feet in toward your pelvis as far as you can comfortably. Let your thighs release down to the mat. Place your fingertips on the mat behind your hips.
- Press into your fingertips and stretch up through your arms. Inhale and press into your buttocks. Elongate your spine all the way to the crown of your head. Exhale fully and lift your upper chest, pressing your shoulder blades together. Remain in this position for several breaths.

Bridge Pose (Setu Bandhasana)

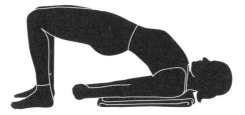

- Lie on your back with your knees bent and your feet flat on the floor, a little wider than hip-width apart. Bend your arms next to your waist, with your palms facing each other. Press your upper arms down to provide extension and length for your ribs.
- Press your feet down as you lift your hips slightly off the floor. Do not extend your pelvis too aggressively.
- As you press your feet down, try to drag your heels up toward your shoulders without actually moving them. This action will contract your hamstrings, lengthen your quadriceps, and keep the strain out of your lower back. Use your hamstrings to help you lift your hips and avoid overstraining your buttocks.
- Breathe for several breaths. Release with a neutral spine.

Cat-Cow

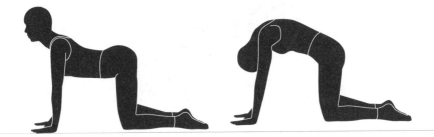

- Start on all fours with your wrists under your shoulders and your knees under your hips. Look forward and lengthen into the crown of your head and into your tailbone. Slightly tip your tailbone up (see Pose 1). Inhale. Press your inner thighs away from each other.
- Exhale and round your spine by curling your chin into your chest and lifting each vertebra up toward the ceiling (see Pose 2). Draw your tailbone in between your legs toward your pubis bone. Your pubis bone should move toward your navel and your navel should recede and press up to the front of your spine. Press your hands down and away from your body as you round your back. Lengthen on the inhalation and round on the exhalation.

Chair Pose (Utkatasana)

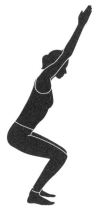

- Stand in Mountain Pose and separate your feet hip-width apart. Bend your hips, knees, and ankles as if to sit down. Ground your feet and slightly draw your weight back into your heels (not onto your back).
- Inhale and press down into your feet as you lower your buttocks and stretch your arms up. Push your hips forward and up, away from your thighs. Your thighs will do most of the work.
- Lengthen into your fingertips while drawing your upper-arm bones back into their socket. Raise your upper chest and rotate your shoulders back toward your spine. Look straight ahead and breathe.
- To come out of the pose, exhale and relax your arms down to your sides as you press your feet into the floor and lift your kneecaps and quadriceps to return to Mountain Pose.

Chair Twist (Bharadvajasana)

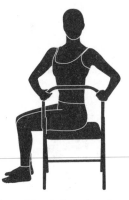

- Sit sideways on a chair. The left side of your body is next to the back of the chair. Plant your feet flat on the floor with your heels under your knees. If your feet do not reach the floor, bring the floor to you by placing a book or two under your feet.
- Hold on to the top of the chair back and bend your elbows wide apart to stretch and open your rib cage. Press your buttocks down into the chair seat as you inhale and lengthen the sides of your body up. Exhale and gradually rotate your body toward the back of the chair. With every inhalation, create lift, extension, and space in your body.
- After 5 breaths, carefully return to center. Repeat on the other side.

Child's Pose (Balasana)

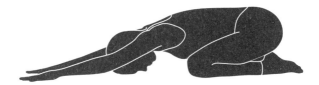

- Start on all fours with your hands under your shoulders and your knees under your hips. Inhale deeply, and then exhale as you draw your buttocks back to rest on your heels.
- Press your hands on your mat, extending into your fingertips, and stretching back through the sides of your body to your hips. Let your forehead rest on the mat. (If your head does not reach the mat, place a folded blanket under your forehead. If your buttocks do not meet your heels, place a folded blanket between your heels and buttocks for support.)
- While in the pose, inhale and feel the expansion of your waist and lower back. Exhale and observe the contraction of your ribs and lungs as the breath leaves your body. Maintain the pose for several breaths and then come back up and release the pose.

Cobra Pose (Bhujangasana)

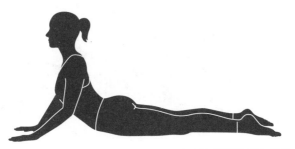

- Lie on your belly with your forehead pointing to the floor, your hands under your shoulders, and your legs outstretched and pressed together behind you. Press your hands and the front of your feet down and lengthen your toes away from your body. Draw your elbows into your waist.
- Inhale and look forward. Stretch your chest, the area between your shoulder blades (upper back), and your ribs forward. Keep your pubic bone on the floor. Exhale.
- Use your hands to press down to lengthen your arms. Your arms do not have to straighten. Breathe!
- Come up only as far as is comfortable. Stay in the pose for a few breaths and then come down.

Downward-Facing Dog
(Adho Mukha Svanasana)

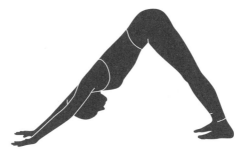

- Start on your hands and knees with your hands under your shoulders and your knees under your hips. Keep your inner arms facing each other and your elbows straight. Let your shoulder blades come together. Keep your pelvis in a neutral position, horizontal to the floor. Tuck your toes under.
- Plant and balance your hands firmly on the floor and spread your fingers evenly apart. Inhale, lift your hips evenly, and press your hands and feet down. On exhalation, straighten your legs and let your head drop down between your arms. Relax your neck. Press the front of your thighs back to elongate your torso. Then stretch your arms away from your hands, all the way up to your buttocks. Let your spine lengthen from the top of your head to your tailbone.
- Remain in the pose for several breaths, extending your spine on inhalation. Then bend your knees and come down.

Eagle Pose (Garudasana)

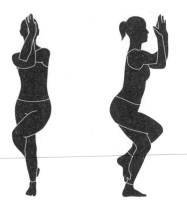

- Stand in Mountain Pose. Extend your arms out to the sides. Bring them to the center and entwine your arms, crossing your left elbow over the inside of your right elbow. Turn your palms to face each other and join them. Lift your elbows to shoulder height and move your forearms away from your face, bringing your wrists over your elbows.
- Bend your hips, knees, and ankles as if you are sitting. Cross your left leg over your right thigh. Press your toes and the balls of your left foot down on the floor. On an exhalation, lift your left foot off the ground and wrap your left shin and foot around your right calf as best you can. Gaze straight ahead.
- Remain in the pose for several breaths and then return to Mountain Pose. Repeat on the other side.

Easy Pose (Sukhasana)

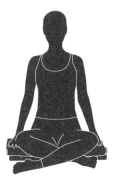

- Sit on one or several folded blankets with your legs crossed. With your hands, roll your inner thighs down to the floor and then ground your buttocks equally as you exhale.
- Inhale, and let your thighs release down to the floor. Lengthen up through the sides of your body. Place your hands by your hips and lift your buttocks off the floor slightly, and then lightly place them back down, maintaining a long torso. Lift and expand your chest. Put your hands palms down on top of your thighs, closer to your hips. Lift and open your upper chest.
- Gaze straight ahead for several breaths. Release the pose, change the cross of your legs, and do the pose again.

Equestrian Pose (Ashwa Sanchalanasana)

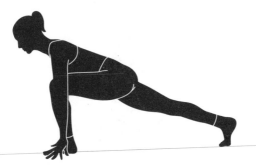

- Come onto all fours. Look forward, bend your left leg, swing it forward, and plant your left foot between your hands. Spread the toes and the balls of your feet and lift your arches. Your left shin should be perpendicular to the floor, with your knee over your heel.
- Extend your right leg from the hip to the heel with your toes tucked under. Lift your back thigh away from the floor slightly to ensure that your thighbone is feeding into the socket. Ground your left foot and the toes of your right foot. Maintain the extension of your spine from the tailbone to the crown of your head. Press your fingertips into the floor as you stretch your arms up into your shoulder sockets to support your upper body.
- Remain in this pose for several breaths. Then release back onto all fours and repeat on the other side.

Extended Hand on the Foot Pose (Utthita Hasta Padangusthasana I)

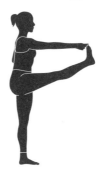

- Stand in Mountain Pose. Transfer your weight onto your left leg and foot. Lift your right leg up and hold it outward, securing your toes with your right hand. (You can also rest your leg on a chair seat or back.) Your outer left hip and ankle should be in line. Stretch both legs fully.
- Try to keep both legs straight by the equal and opposite reactions of pressing into your feet, lifting your arches and fully stretching up through your legs, lifting your kneecaps, contracting your quadriceps muscles, and hugging your thigh muscles into the bone. Do not lock your knees. Stretch your whole body up. Try to keep your buttocks level with each other.
- Remain in this pose for a few breaths. On the exhalation, bring your arms and leg down. Repeat on the other side.

Extended Side Angle Pose
(Utthita Parsvakonasana)

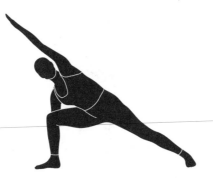

- Start in Mountain Pose and move your legs apart as wide as you can comfortably. Turn your left foot in 15 degrees and revolve your right leg out. Keep your heels in line with each other. Ground your feet, spread your toes, and lift your arches.
- Inhale through your nostrils and lengthen up through your legs and the sides of your body. Exhale fully as you bend your right leg (at the hip, knee, and ankle), with your knee in line with your heel. Your leg will form a 90-degree angle. Bend at your hip, directly to the side over your right leg, and bring your right hand behind your right foot, with your fingertips touching the ground. Inhale and extend your

left arm up and over your head. Lengthen up the left side of your body into your fingertips. Look straight ahead with your chest facing forward, keeping your head in line with your spine. Stretch into the crown of your head and into your tailbone. Continue breathing naturally.

- Stay in this pose for a few breaths. Turn your feet back to parallel, and then repeat on the other side.

Four-Limbed Staff Pose
(Chattaranga Dandasana)

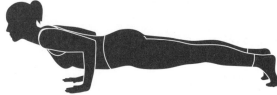

- Lie down on your belly with your legs extended and your hands under your shoulders, fingers facing forward. Your elbows should be next to your waist. Press your hands down and lift the top of your shoulders away from the floor. The goal is to have your shoulders at the same height as your elbows throughout the pose.
- Shrug your shoulders toward your ears slightly to feed the upper-arm bones into the shoulder sockets. Tuck the toes way under and walk them toward your body. Your thighbones insert into their hip sockets, supporting your pelvis. Now stretch your heels away from the back of your body to stretch your legs from hamstrings to heels. Feel your thighs and hips lift slightly off the floor.
- Inhale and as you exhale, lift your body off the floor. Your hips and shoulders should be at the same height off the floor. Stay up for a second and then come down. Use your breath to facilitate the movement into the pose.

Half-Moon Pose (Ardha Chandrasana)

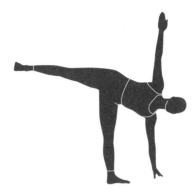

- To begin, stand in Mountain Pose. Walk your feet wide apart. Turn your left foot in 15 degrees and revolve your right leg out. Inhale and lift your ribs, and then on the exhalation, come into Triangle Pose.
- As you reach up with your right hand, bend your right leg to a right angle and place the fingertips of your left hand firmly on the floor, several inches in front of your left foot. Walk your back leg toward the front. If your fingers do not reach the floor, use a block to bring the floor to you.
- Press into your right foot, stretching your leg fully, and draw your standing leg muscles up to the hip socket. At the same time, lift your left leg up parallel to the floor. Pull up the standing leg kneecap. Extend through your left heel and balls of your foot to maintain energy and firmness in your leg. Repeat on the other side.

Head-to-Knee Pose (Janu Sirsasana)

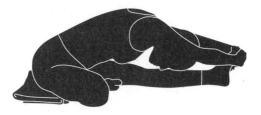

- Sit evenly on your buttocks with your legs outstretched and together in front of you. Bend your right leg out to the side. Holding on to the back of your knee, draw your knee back to a comfortable position. Place the sole of your foot by your inner thigh. Your left leg should be extended, with the center of your back heel on the floor. Your left foot is actively spreading, inner and outer arches are lifting, and the balls, joints of your toes, and heel are stretching forward.
- Turn your body to face your left leg. Clasp your outer foot or hold on to your outer shin with your hands. Turn your navel to face your inner left leg. Press down evenly with your buttocks, the back of your left leg, and your right thigh. Lengthen up through the sides of your body. Draw your upper-arm bones back into their sockets.

- Make your back concave, creating more length in your spine. Inhale, and on exhalation, bend from your hips and extend your body out over your extended left leg. Repeat on the other side.

Intense Side Stretch Pose (Parsvottanasana)

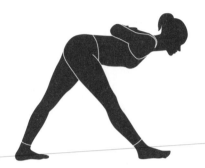

- Stand in Mountain Pose. Jump or walk your feet wide apart. Place your hands on your hips. Turn your left foot in 45–60 degrees, and turn your right leg out. Inhale, ground your feet, lift your arches, and bring the inhalation and extension all the way up your legs and body.
- Exhale and turn to face your right leg. Place your hands in reverse prayer position behind the middle of your back. Revolve your left leg in its socket, turning your front thigh to face forward (without strain or force). Inhale and extend your spine, looking up. Exhale and, bending from the hips, swing your body over your right leg. Gaze at your toes. Lengthen from the crown of your head to your tailbone.
- See if you can balance the forward action of your torso extending over your front leg by pulling your hips back and drawing the tops

of your thighs and your hamstrings behind you. If you can bend more deeply in your hips and maintain the length created in your spine, bring your head toward your shin.

- Simultaneously level your hips by pulling your outer right hip back and releasing your left hip forward to help you turn your hips even more. Stay in the pose for a few breaths. Repeat on the other side. Place your back heel on the wall if you need additional support.

Locust Pose (Salabhasana)

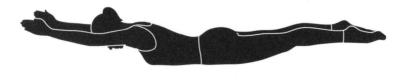

- Lie on your belly with your legs together and extended. Stretch into your toes. Reach your arms out in front of you on the mat with your palms facing each other. Stretch into your fingertips. Inhale, and then exhale as you firm your abdominals.
- Keeping your abdominals firm, inhale, lift, and extend your arms and legs. Keep breathing and lengthening into your fingers and toes. Your head should be between your arms and lifted up at the same height.
- After several breaths exhale and release the pose. Rest on your belly with your head to the side.

Mountain Pose (Tadasana)

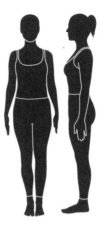

- Place your feet together. Stand so your ankles, knees, and hips are lined up, one over the other. When viewed from one side, your ear, shoulder, hip, knee, and ankle should form a straight vertical line, with your arms by your sides.
- Spread the toes and balls of your feet, pressing into the big and little toe mounds and the center of your heels. Bring your weight a little more into your heels. Lift your arches as you ground your feet. Lengthen your leg muscles all the way up to your hips. Lift the tops of your kneecaps by contracting your quadriceps. Place your hands on your hips and extend the sides of your body from your hips to your armpits.

- Bring your arms back to your sides without losing the lift of the spine and lengthen up through the crown of your head. Balance your head over your pelvis. Relax your shoulders. Press your shoulder blades into your back. Broaden your collarbones. Breathe.

Pigeon Pose (Raja Kapotasana Modified)

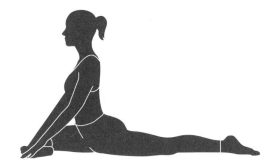

- Start on all fours. Bring your right leg through as in the Equestrian Pose. Once your right foot is between your hands, let the right side of your leg rest on the floor. The outside of your right shin and thigh will be against the floor. Your fingertips will be on either side of your right leg. Adjust the angles of your right leg so you are comfortable. Tuck the toes of your back leg under to provide more muscle energy in your back leg. Try to balance your weight between your legs by rolling more onto the straight (back) leg.
- Prop yourself up on your arms by placing the fingertips of each hand on the floor, stretching up through your arms and spine. Let your hips sink down as if you were sitting. Stretch into your back heel. Remain in this pose for several breaths. Then come back onto all fours and repeat on the other side.

Plank Pose (Phalakasana)

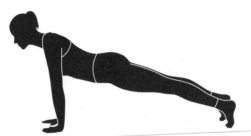

- Lie down on your belly, bend your arms, and place your hands on the floor and under your shoulders (fingers facing forward). Extend your legs behind you and tuck your toes under.
- Press your hands down firmly and feel your upper-back muscles start contracting and drawing in to your shoulder blades and against your back.
- Press your hands and toes down, exhale, and stretch your arms up into your shoulder sockets, lifting your torso and legs off the floor. Make sure your shoulder blades are supporting and opening your chest. Stretch your heels away from your body as the front of your thighs firm and stretch.
- Remain in this pose for several breaths and then come down.

Reclining Hand-to-Big-Toe Pose I (Supta Padangusthasana I)

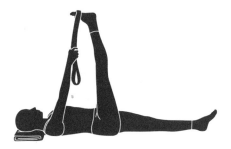

- Lie down and extend your legs on the floor. Extend your right leg up, with the sole of your foot facing the ceiling. Hold on to your big toe with your first two fingers, hold on to the outside of your foot, or use a strap to hold your toes.
- Press the back of your left leg down. Lengthen your inner and outer heels away from your ankles, spread your toes, and lift your inner and outer arches.
- Elongate the sides of your body from your hips to your armpits. Lengthen from your right waist to your hip to equalize both sides of your body. (Your right side will want to shorten because of your leg being raised.)
- Stay in this pose for several breaths and then lower your leg and repeat on the other side.

Reclining Hand-to-Big-Toe Pose II
(Supta Padangusthasana II)

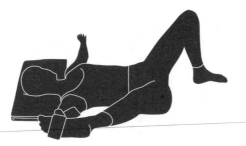

- Lie down and raise your right leg perpendicularly. Place a belt around the outstretched leg and hold on to the strap with the same hand as the raised leg. Bend your bottom leg with your foot flat on the floor to make it more comfortable for your hamstrings. Place your bottom foot against a wall for enhanced stretching of the bottom leg. Fully stretch your legs throughout the pose.
- On an exhalation, lower your right leg down to the right side. Your hips must remain level with each other, so your leg may not reach the floor. Look at the ceiling.
- Remain in this pose for a few breaths and then carefully raise your leg back up perpendicularly, release it, and lower your leg to the floor. Repeat on the other side.

Reclining Hero Pose (Supta Virasana)

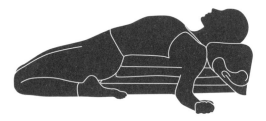

- Come to a kneeling position. Place two to four vertically folded blankets, one on top of the other, behind your buttocks. Sit down evenly between your feet. Your feet should touch each hip (as best you can). Pressing down into your buttocks, exhale, inhale, and lengthen up through your spine to the crown of your head. Stretch and spread your toes and the soles of your feet. Place your hands palms down on either side of the blankets and lengthen your spine out of your pelvis. Rest on your elbows as your body lowers onto the blankets.
- Remain in this pose up to 5 minutes, depending upon your level of comfort and ease. This is another great restorative pose. To come out of the pose, press your elbows and forearms down on either side of the blankets and come up with your chest lifted. Carefully extend one leg at a time.

Restorative Bridge Pose
(Setu Bandhasana Sarvangasana)

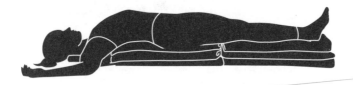

- Place two bolsters vertically, one behind the other (or use four to six blankets vertically folded) on the floor. Lie down with your whole body and legs on the bolsters, so the bottom edge of your shoulder blades are on the upper edge of the top bolster. The tops of your shoulders should roll down to the floor, doming and expanding your upper chest. The back of your head should also be on the floor. Your arms can rest horizontally by your sides, with your palms facing up, or they can be bent at the elbows, like a cactus. Keep your elbows in line with your shoulders.
- Loop a belt firmly around the middle of your thighs so they will not be able to roll apart. An extra belt can also be looped around the middle of your shins for extra support.

- Close your eyes and relax. Remain in this pose from 5–15 minutes. To come out of the pose, bend your knees with your feet flat on the floor, and release the belt. Then carefully roll onto your right side with your knees bent and use your hands to bring yourself up to a seated position.

Revolved Side Angle Pose
(Parivritta Parsvakonasana)

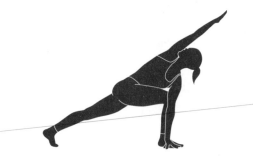

- Begin by standing in Mountain Pose. Walk your feet wide apart. Extend your arms from your heart to your fingertips. Turn your left foot in 45–60 degrees. Turn your right leg out so your foot is at 90 degrees. Inhale, and on exhalation, turn to face your front (right) leg. Inhale and extend up from your feet into your fingertips. Exhale and bend your right leg. Bend forward from your hips and turn your whole body to face your right leg.

- Press your left fingertips down on the floor by the outside of your right foot and extend your arm. Place your right palm on the small of your back. Lengthen your spine as you inhale and further rotate your body around your spine as you exhale. Keep your head in line with your spine. When ready, extend your right arm up and over your head.

- Breathe. On an exhale, bring your feet parallel, center your body, and release your arms down to your sides. Repeat on the other side.

Revolved Triangle Pose (Parivritta Trikonasana)

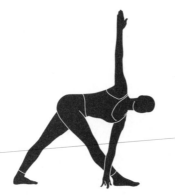

- Stand in Mountain Pose and walk your legs wide apart. Inhale and extend your arms out to your sides. Turn your left foot in 45–60 degrees and rotate your right leg out so your foot is at 90 degrees.
- On an exhalation, turn your body to face your right leg. Revolve your back (left) leg so the front of your thigh faces forward. Turn toward the right as you extend your torso, and place your left hand on the mat by the outside of your right foot. Place your right palm on your lower back. Continue revolving your torso around the axis of your spine as you extend from the crown of your head to your tailbone. Extend your right arm up, stretching into your fingertips. Contract your leg muscles firmly.
- Inhale, and come up out of the pose slowly. Turn your feet back to parallel and center your body. Repeat on the other side.

Sage Twist (Maricyasana III)

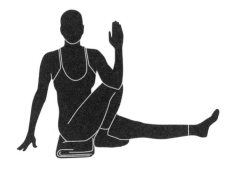

- Sit evenly on your buttocks with your legs extended and together in front of you (place a folded blanket under your buttocks if it is more comfortable). Lengthen your arms and torso. Bring your right knee to your chest and your heel to your right buttock. Firmly plant your right foot. Extend through your left leg and press the back of your leg down.
- Turn to the right. Wrap your left arm around your right knee and hug your leg into your body, pressing the fingertips of your right hand into the mat behind you.
- Inhale, extend your left arm up, and exhale as you bring the outside of your arm against the outside of your bent right knee. Press your arm against your leg as leverage to help with the rotation of the

twist. Inhale and extend your spine. Exhale and spiral your torso toward your right leg. Move your right knee forward and bring your back ribs into your front ribs. Stretch your fingertips up to deepen the action and bring your shoulder blades toward your back.

- Do this for several breaths, gently increasing the rotation of your spine and torso. Slowly release, and repeat on the other side.

Salute with Eight Parts or Points
(Ashtanga Namaskara)

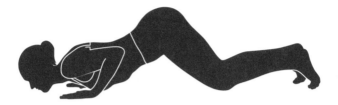

- Begin in Plank Pose. Exhale and extend down into your heels, rebounding down into your feet and hands to move up, stretching your sternum forward and keeping your legs and abdominals firm. Keep your shoulders over your wrists with your hands on the floor.
- Inhale. Exhale and lower your knees, chest, and chin to the mat.

Seated Straight-Leg Forward Bend
(Paschimottanasana)

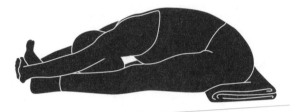

- Sit evenly on your buttocks with your legs extended and together in front of you. Press your fingertips down on either side as you lengthen up through the sides of your torso. Clasp your feet with both hands. Ground your buttocks and the backs of your legs. Draw your thighbones back into their hip sockets.
- Inhale, look up, and lift up through the crown of your head, creating a concave spine. Exhale as you bend forward from your hips and extend your body over your legs. Lift your ribs away from your hips.
- Remain in this pose for several breaths. See if you can create more internal space as you inhale, and move deeper into the pose (if appropriate) with each exhale. Inhale up the front of your spine and exhale down the back. Your forehead can rest on your legs or remain extended in the air.

Seated Wide-Angle Pose (Upavistha Konasana)

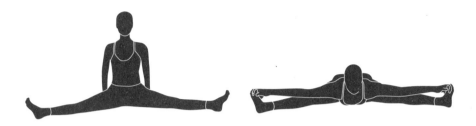

- Sit evenly on your buttocks with your legs extended in front of you. Separate your legs as far apart as you can comfortably. Press your fingertips down by the sides of your body to lift and elongate your torso. Lift your rib cage off your hips. Root the center of the back of your heels and legs into the floor. Your toes should face the ceiling. Breathe.
- To go further into the pose, bend forward from your hips and extend your body out and forward. Maintain the elongation of the front, sides, and back of your body. Grasp your big toes or calves with your hands. Keeps your buttocks grounded on the floor. Lower your head to the floor if you like.

Sideways Wide-Angle Pose
(Parsva Upavistha Konasana)

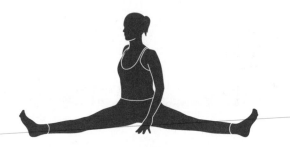

- Sit in Seated Wide-Angle Pose. Place your right fingertips behind you and your left fingertips on the floor in front of your pubis. Press your fingertips down and ground your legs and buttocks as you inhale and lift your spine and the sides of your body.
- Exhale and gently rotate your body toward your right leg. Do this for several breaths, gently increasing the rotation of your spine and torso. Then carefully unwind back to center. Repeat on the other side.

Sphinx Pose

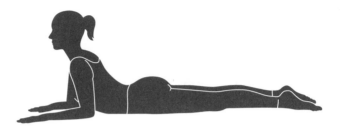

- Lie on your belly with your legs extended behind you. Prop yourself up on your forearms. Your forearms will be parallel to each other with your elbows close to your waist and in line with your wrists and shoulders. Press your forearms and palms down and lift your chest, elongating the sides of your body.
- Pull your elbows back on the floor without actually moving them. Feel the muscles of your upper back draw into your back and hug your shoulder blades. Lift your sternum forward and up.
- Remain in this pose for several breaths and then release and rest.

Standing Backbend Pose (Anuvittasana)

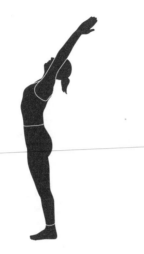

- Stand in Mountain Pose with your feet hip-width apart. Ground your feet and contract your thighs. Inhale, extend your spine and arms forward, and raise yourself with a concave back and long legs.
- Raise your arms over your head, look up, lift your heart, and arch your back. Exhale and return to Mountain Pose.

Standing Forward Bend (Uttanasana)

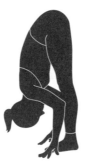

- Stand in Mountain Pose. Inhale, root down onto your feet, and elongate your spine as you contract your kneecaps and quadriceps. Lift up through your crown.
- Roll your upper inner thighs and groin muscles back, keeping your lower back broad. Draw your shoulder blades into your back to lift and open your chest. Lift and stretch your sides and spine up and over as you exhale and bend forward, folding at your hips.
- Place your fingertips on the floor in front of your feet (or bend down as far as you can comfortably). Breathe and allow the effects of gravity to release your back muscles and spine, with your head down. Contract your quadriceps to lengthen your hamstrings.
- When you are ready to come up, press your feet down and let your thigh muscles support your hamstring and prevent hyperextension of the knees. Look forward, inhale, and come up with a concave back.

Standing Half-Forward Bend (Ardha Uttanasana)

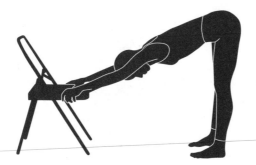

- Stand in front of a chair. Bend over to place your hands on the sides of the chair seat and press your hands into the seat. Stretch your arms back into their shoulder sockets.
- Keep your elbows firm and straight. Continue lengthening from your shoulders to your buttocks, making the sides of your waist long. Keep your chest open and your spine long.
- Keep your neck and head in line with your spine. Stretch the crown of your head forward as your tailbone lengthens back. Keep your heels in line with your buttocks and your feet hip-width (or wider) apart. Ground your feet and contract your leg muscles.

Supported Bound Angle Pose
(Supta Baddha Konasana)

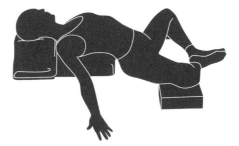

- Stack one to three vertically folded blankets behind you, with the narrow end a few inches away from your buttocks. Sit evenly on your buttocks with your legs extended and together in front of you. Bend your knees out to the sides and join the soles of your feet together. Draw your heels in toward your pelvis as far as you can comfortably.
- Place your hands on either side of the blankets and lower your back (keeping it extended) and head onto the blankets. Let your arms come out to the sides, with your palms facing up. Close your eyes. Relax and breathe.
- To come out of the pose, bring your knees together and carefully roll off the blankets onto your right side. Bring yourself to a seated position.

Supported Legs Up the Wall Pose
(Viparita Karani)

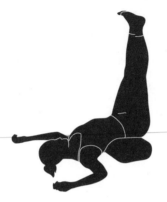

- Place a bolster or one to three horizontally folded blankets against a wall. Lie on your side with your left hip on the support, buttocks close to the wall, and knees bent. Roll onto your back and swing your legs up the wall. Rest your legs on the wall with your lower back and sacrum on the support and the rest of your torso on the mat. Raise your arms to the sides of your head with your elbows bent and your palms up. The eyes may close and soften.
- Breathe naturally. To come out of the pose, bend your knees and roll over onto your right side. Use your hands to press yourself up into a seated position.

Supported Shoulderstand
(Salamba Sarvangasana)

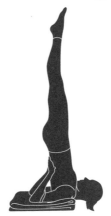

- Stack three folded blankets on top of each other, rounded edges together and facing away from the wall, a foot or so away from the wall. Lie down on the blankets with your neck off the top edges. Place your feet on the wall with your knees bent (adjust your distance to the wall so your legs can be at 90 degrees).
- Bend your elbows and press your upper arms down, and as you inhale lift your buttocks. Support your lower back with your hands. Keep your head on the floor, your shoulders on the blankets, and your neck slightly off the floor.

- As your upper arms press down, allow your body and legs to extend up. Press your shoulder blades into your back, opening your chest and drawing your upper spine into your body. Use your hands to support your torso, but use your back muscles, your legs, and your pelvis to hold you up in this pose.
- Remain in this pose for several breaths, keeping your throat soft, then release your hands from your back and slowly lower to the ground.

Tree Pose I (Vrksasana I)

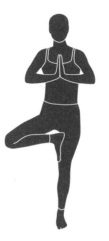

- Stand in Mountain Pose. Gaze straight ahead. Shift your weight to your left leg and press down firmly with your entire foot, from your toes to your heel.
- Bring your right foot up to the inside of your left leg to where it is comfortable. Maintain the grounding in your left foot and the extension in your left leg, taking care not to hyperextend your leg.
- Press your palms together at your heart center.

Tree Pose II (Vrksasana II)

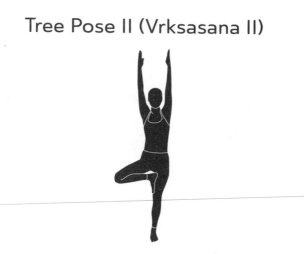

- Stand in Mountain Pose. Gaze straight ahead. Shift your weight to your left leg and press down firmly with your entire foot, from your toes to your heel.
- Bring your right foot up to the inside of your left leg to where it is comfortable. Maintain the grounding in your left foot and the extension in your left leg, taking care not to hyperextend your leg.
- Extend your arms out to your sides with your palms facing up. Stretch all the way from the centerline of your body to your fingertips. On an inhalation, bring your arms up over your head, stretching from your sides to your fingertips, palms facing each other. Continue breathing. Remain in this pose for several breaths, and then repeat on the other side.

Triangle Pose (Utthita Trikonasana)

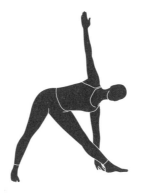

- Stand in Mountain Pose. Walk your feet apart as far as you can comfortably and actively stretch your arms up through your fingertips. Feel the opening of your chest and upper ribs. Turn your right foot in 15 degrees and rotate your left leg out. Your left foot should be at about a 120-degree angle to your right foot, with your left and right heels in line with each other.
- Inhale and lengthen up through your legs. Contract your quadriceps. Exhale and extend laterally over your left leg, bending from the hip.
- Lower your left arm and place your fingertips lightly on your left shin or on the floor. Raise your right arm straight up, working to stack your shoulders. Keep your head in line with your spine

and lengthen from the crown of your head to your tailbone. Look straight ahead.

- Maintain the pose for several breaths. Breathe normally. Inhale, release your arms to your sides, and bring your feet parallel. Repeat on the other side.

Upward-Facing Dog (Urdhva Mukha Svanasana)

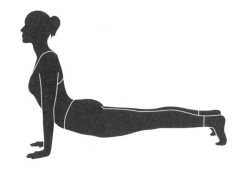

- Lie down on your belly. Extend your legs straight out behind you. Place your hands flat on the mat by your waist, fingers facing forward. Stretch from your legs to your toes; contract your thigh muscles. Inhale and look forward. Extend your chest and your upper back forward and your ribs forward and up.
- Press your hands and feet down to lift your legs slightly off the floor and to support your torso. Exhale and stretch into your toes as you continue coiling your spine forward and up. Bring your upper arms back and open your upper chest to draw your shoulder blades in toward your back. Lift your kneecaps and firm your thighs.
- Remain in this pose for several breaths and then come down and release.

Warrior I (Virabhadrasana I)

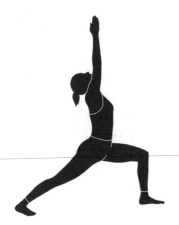

- Stand in Mountain Pose. Jump or walk your legs a few feet apart. Extend your arms out to your sides, palms facing up. Stretch into your fingertips and feel the opening of your chest and ribs. Inhale and lift your arms up over your head.
- Stretch your side ribs by lifting your arms. Keep your palms facing each other, lengthen your arms, and firm your elbows.
- Turn your right foot in 45–60 degrees and rotate your left leg out. On an exhalation, turn your body to face your front (left) leg. Ground through your feet, lift your arches, and extend all the way from your feet to your legs, through your body, and into your fingertips. Relax the top of your shoulders away from your ears.

- Inhale, then as you exhale, bend your left leg and lengthen your right leg, pressing the top of your right thigh back. Bend your left leg to create a right angle.
- Remain in this pose for a few breaths. Repeat on the other side.

Warrior II (Virabhadrasana II)

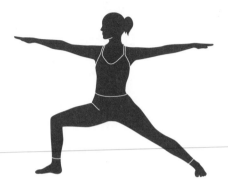

- Inhale and walk your feet wide apart. Lift and extend your arms out to the sides from the center of your body to your fingertips throughout the pose. Open and lift your chest as you inhale. Turn your left foot in 15 degrees and rotate your right leg out 90 degrees, heel in line with heel. Press your feet firmly down.
- Inhale, then exhale fully and bend your right leg to a 90-degree angle with your knee over your ankle. (If you cannot get into a 90-degree angle, just do the best you can without strain.) As you bend your right leg, keep your left leg long and grounded. Contract your quadriceps. Keep your body centered between your legs.
- To come out of the pose, press down into your right foot, lift your kneecap and thigh to lengthen your right leg, and turn your feet parallel. Repeat on the other side.

Wide-Legged Forward Bend
(Prasarita Padottanasana)

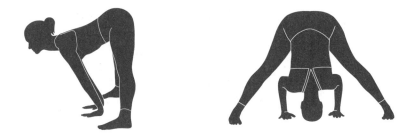

- Stand in Mountain Pose and walk your feet wide apart, parallel to each other. Press the soles of your feet down. Firm your quadriceps. Press your shoulder blades into your back to open and lift your chest. Breathe and expand your lungs out to your side ribs.
- Inhale. As you exhale, fold forward from the hips, maintaining the length of your spine. Place your fingertips on the floor (or your palms, if flexible), shoulder-width apart, either in line with your toes or in front of them.
- Look straight ahead. Keep breathing, and on an exhalation, fold deeper into the hip if possible. Remain in this pose for a few breaths.
- Bend down further and let your head hang down. Rise on an inhale with a flat back and your arms extended to your sides.

INDEX